Care of the
Dying Patient

JUN   2010

Care of the
Dying Patient

Edited by David A. Fleming and John C. Hagan III

University of Missouri Press
Columbia and London

Copyright © 2010 by
The Curators of the University of Missouri
University of Missouri Press, Columbia, Missouri 65201
Printed and bound in the United States of America
All rights reserved
5 4 3 2 1   14 13 12 11 10

Cataloging-in-Publication data available from the Library of Congress
ISBN 978-0-8262-1874-2 (cloth) 978-0-8262-1890-2 (paper)

∞™ This paper meets the requirements of the
American National Standard for Permanence of Paper
for Printed Library Materials, Z39.48, 1984.

Design and composition: Aaron Lueders
Printing and binding: Integrated Book Technology Inc.
Typefaces: Palatino, Myriad Pro, Futura

This book is dedicated to my parents, Dr. J. Will and Mary Louise Fleming, whose gifts of wisdom and caring illuminated my path as a physician.

—David A. Fleming

Contents

Part 1: Control of Suffering

Part 2: The Needs of Special Populations

Part 3: Psychological and Spiritual Needs

Foreword

For centuries, care of the dying was an occasion for compassion, empathy, ritual, and prayer, not an exercise in ethical decision making. Most cultures possessed customs, symbols, and religious practices designed to provide comfort and solace to dying people and their families. Any decisions made centered on nonmedical issues, such as succession to the dying person's social role, power, wealth, or possessions. Physicians attended mainly to relieve pain and to make the official pronouncement of death.

All of this has changed drastically in the last half century. Ethical decisions now dominate what formerly was a time of community solicitude. Discord between and among families, physicians, and other health-care professionals is now common. Dissent about divergent potential courses of action in a dying patient's care constitutes the most frequent reason for ethics consultations. Everyone sincerely wants to do the right and good thing—especially when the patient loses the capacity to voice his or her opinion of what that means. But deciding what is right and good has become vastly more complicated than before due to three overarching changes in our society: the expanded power of medical biotechnology over all phases of human life, the proliferating diversity of cultural and religious belief systems, and the rise of participatory democracy, predominantly, though not exclusively, in Western societies.

Of these three, the precipitating factor is the power of physicians to determine the manner, timing, and quality

of dying virtually at will. As a result, the natural history of
every disease has been radically altered. The life of the dis-
eased person can be lengthened or shortened, and its quality
shaped by cultural, religious, personal, and social determinants. Life-sustaining treatments can enhance or impede
nonmedical ends, and choices must be made.

At one time, at least in circumscribed communities,
there might have been uniformity in the values underlying such decisions. This is very rarely the case today. Much
more frequently, the assemblage of decision makers—
physicians, nurses, social workers, pastoral counselors, family members, and patient—will differ among themselves on
the most fundamental questions: What is the meaning and
value of human life? What constitutes a "quality life"? Is assisted suicide or euthanasia morally permissible?

Added to the power of biotechnology and the complexities of moral diversity is the growing power of patients and
surrogates to participate in clinical decisions. From merely
the right to refuse treatment, the autonomy rights of patients
or their surrogates have expanded to become a virtual right
to demand and in some cases to micromanage treatment. On
principle, each person in the decision-making assemblage,
as a human being, is owed respect for his or her person and
dignity. Health professionals cannot impose their notion of
what is good on the patient or his or her surrogates. Neither can patients or their surrogates impose their will on
the health professional. Nor can one health professional, for
example, the physician, impose his or her will on the other,
for example, the nurse.

In the midst of this potpourri of values, demands, and
obligations, there is often some "advance directive" which
formally or informally purports to represent what the patient would want, could the patient make his or her own
decision. Anyone who has tried to interpret a living will in
the face of the conflicting interpretations of what that will
means at the actual moment of decision making knows how
troubling an advance directive can be.

The number of books and articles end-of-life ethics has generated is overwhelming, but the current volume has several things to recommend it even in the face of such a surfeit of advice now available. For one thing, this book more closely articulates hospice and palliative care with the end-of-life decision-making process. Secondly, the essays here derive from a successful series of articles in *Missouri Medicine*; no state has seen more discussion of these issues than Missouri. In 1989, the historic and unfortunate right-to-die case of Nancy Cruzan went from Missouri to the United States Supreme Court and ended there. Finally, this book covers all dimensions of this matter, legal and medical, in an integrated and effective way.

Nearly every one of us, sooner or later, must face these decisions for ourselves or for members of our families. Many will be in the position of serving as surrogate decision makers, holding the authority of a durable power of attorney for health or in an unofficial position when no advance directive exists. No one can responsibly afford to be ignorant of these complex issues and the inescapable necessity for making a decision under these conditions.

Medicine's advances are creating ethical issues because they afford many more choices than ever before about how long we live and how our lives end. More medical advances are sure to come and more dilemmas sure to follow. If participatory democracy is to be a viable reality, bioethics must become everybody's business. This book will assist that aim at least in providing discussion of the most frequently encountered ethical decisions we will all face one day.

Edmund D. Pellegrino, MD, MACP

Acknowledgments

Many thanks go to our able assistant, Adam Desaulniers, in the final assembly of this text before submission to the publisher. We also wish to recognize that this manuscript is, in great part, a compilation of revised essays reprinted with permission from *Missouri Medicine* 2002 Nov/Dec;99(6), Copyright 2002, and 2003 Jan/Feb;100(1), Copyright 2003, Missouri State Medical Association. We also have permission to reprint the revised essay by Debra Parker Oliver, "Redefining Hope for the Terminally Ill," which originally appeared in the *American Journal of Hospice and Palliative Medicine* 2002;19(2):115–121, Copyright 2002, Prime National Publishing Corp.

Care of the
Dying Patient

Introduction

David A. Fleming and John C. Hagan III

More than two million Americans die every year. Health-care providers are therefore forced daily to confront often agonizing decisions that must be made for dying patients. Patients and their families face difficult choices about the "quality of death" that dying will have and the kind of care they need and want at the end of life. Though death can be dramatically delayed by the ever expanding capabilities of medical technology, ultimately, death cannot be indefinitely postponed. Unfortunately, the culture of medicine has been slow to accept this reality. Physicians and family often reluctantly and belatedly accept death when further treatment is irrefutably futile. This delay in acceptance tends to delay referral to hospice and palliative-care services at a time when dying patients need them the most. In addition, when death is imminent, physicians may be prone to withdraw from their patients, feeling that their skills of diagnosis and treatment have failed and they are no longer needed or wanted. Paradoxically, trust and ongoing commitment by physicians to *care* for patients are never more important, or more needed, than when death looms.

Over the past several years patients and health-care providers both have recognized these concerns and are developing greater understanding about death and dying. Physicians are now learning the importance of knowing and respecting the wishes of their patients, and they are optimizing care at the end of life, even when further treatment is futile in terms of prolonging life. The American Medical Association's 1995 Study to Understand Prognosis and Preferences for Outcomes and Risks of Treatments (SUPPORT) documented that dying in this country is unnecessarily painful and costly and that physicians often do not understand or respond to patients' wishes. In 1997 the Institute of Medicine reported, "People have come to fear a technologically over-treated and protracted death and dread the prospect of abandonment and untreated physical and emotional stress." In 1996 the Robert Wood Johnson Foundation launched "Last Acts," a national campaign to promote improvements in care of patients near the end of life. This initiative has promoted changes in health policy and communication with health-care providers and consumer groups about the need to optimize end-of-life care. The Last Acts campaign is working to ensure that seriously ill and dying patients receive the best care available and have the fullest understanding possible about the options available to them. Collectively, these are "quality-of-death" issues.

In attempting to address these pressing concerns, the authors of this text offer a series of writings, many of which were originally published as a series of acclaimed articles in the *Missouri Medicine* medical journal, to further elucidate the issues and offer solutions to providers, patients, families, and caregivers confronted by incurable illness and death. All physicians and care providers must learn that relieving pain and physical suffering, though important and a major challenge, is not the only concern when caring for dying patients. Providers should also know when and how to effectively utilize palliative-care services and to refer patients to hospice in a timely manner. Though increasingly important, these concepts are still poorly understood. All must learn to be responsive to the needs of our patients resulting from their cultural and spiritual or religious beliefs and remain sensitive to the differences that exist in these areas. Physicians and other providers must also be prepared to address the often agonizing forms of spiritual and psychological suffering that dying patients endure, including the loss of hope that often overshadows physical suffering. We also address the burden of caregiving that is typically provided by untrained family members. This must be considered by the health-care team as caregivers become increasingly involved in the coordinated care and treatment of their loved ones near the end of life. Caregiving is an increasingly important concern and extends well beyond the care of patients with cancer. The United States and most developed countries have aging populations with an exponential growth of patients diagnosed with Alzheimer's disease. This is a major consideration in addressing the allocation of health-care resources and the compelling challenge that physicians have to help older patients and their families make end-of-life decisions. As our country ages, we will have an ever-larger number of patients with cancer and other forms of terminal illness. This means that nonprofessional, nonpaid (usually family) caregiving will become increasingly important in the overall scheme of end-of-life care. The risks and stresses involved in caregiving have huge implications for the overall success of end-of-life care and how the trust relationship develops between physician, patient, and caregivers.

This book emphasizes palliative care and hospice care because physicians are often reluctant to refer patients to these programs for fear that doing so will be viewed as abandonment. Physicians also resist using opioids and other controlled substances aggressively for dying patients; this resistance may stem from a poor understanding about indications for these drugs and fear of retribution from regulatory agencies for using them. In addition, physicians may have strongly held personal beliefs about performing actions that may lead to premature death. We, as physicians, are both ethically and legally accountable for our actions. However, physicians should not be afraid to act according to the needs of their patients, even if that means aggressively using opioids or other controlled substances or withdrawing futile treatment when indicated.

Referenced in some of our chapters is a major contribution from the American Medical Association, the Education in Palliative and End-of-Life Care (EPEC) Project (originally called Education for Physicians in End-of-Life Care), which was developed in 1999 to help bridge the gap between patient/family expectations and the current state of end-of-life care. The goals of EPEC are to help physicians and other health-care providers develop the skills and confidence that will enable them to provide good end-of-life care, to strengthen physician-patient relationships, and to enhance physicians' personal satisfaction with the interaction and care they provide patients and their caregivers.

EPEC is a modulated program with four plenary presentations and seventeen modules that cover a wide range of clinical decision making and the basic concepts of interdisciplinary supportive care. Though EPEC is not an attempt to make every physician an expert in palliative care, it will enable greater competence through skill building and enhance confidence of physicians who face the difficult and challenging circumstances of suffering and dying. The psychological and physical symptoms that accompany death can be severe, often dramatically affecting patients' will to live and their sense of autonomy. Although treatment for even the most severe forms of cancer pain is available and can be effective if done with an informed, multidisciplinary approach, surprisingly, up to one-half of patients in programs devoted to palliative care still report significant pain one week before death.

The barriers to and pitfalls of effective end-of-life care may be daunting, but they are not insurmountable. The means to provide effective relief of suffering and to optimize the quality of death of terminally ill patients, their families, and their caregivers are available and can be accessed through the resources provided in this text and through referral to specialists in palliative-care and hospice services. As the needs and expectations of patients and their families become more challenging with the progression of disease, and as effective treatments diminish in the march toward death, the opportunities for providing care instead of treatment become more compelling. We hope this text will be a helpful resource for students and learners in the health professions, and for all students preparing for participation in the health-care team as members of the clergy or in social work.

Through building their skills, increasing their awareness, and fine tuning their insight, physicians and other health-care providers have the opportunity to develop the ability to meet the needs and expectations of patients and their families through trusting, caring, and committed relationships. Optimal communication, good documentation, informed decision making (by both physicians and patients), and fearless use of interventions that will relieve suffering of all forms are the keys to success in end-of-life care. Effectively integrating these components for the benefit of patients in the future will be the ultimate challenge in the always-changing environment of health care. This text is presented in the belief that everyone should experience the highest possible quality of death.

Part 1
Control of Suffering

1
Pain Management at the End of Life
Clay M. Anderson

Pain is a universal aspect of life and part of our sensory experience. It is necessary and adaptive. At the same time, it is a form of suffering that can affect the duration and detract from the quality of human life. Currently, there are both pharmacologic and nonpharmacologic tools that allow us to modify pain in such a way as to minimize its impact on quality of life. This is a miracle of modern medicine. Still, around the world as well as in the United States, most pain sufferers are inadequately treated, for a variety of reasons.[1] In other countries, the necessary medications may not be available.[2] In the United States, the barriers to adequate pain modification include regulatory burdens, cost, myths about pain and pain medicines, and lack of education for the public and for medical professionals.[3]

Significant pain is present in the majority of patients dying of chronic diseases such as cancer, heart disease, lung disease, and diabetes.[4] End-of-life care entails treating patients with these chronic diseases when the diseases are in their final phase, with the focus on bringing about relief of suffering and aggressively treating symptoms caused by the diseases. The common complaint of pain at the end of life is usually eminently treatable now, yet most patients remain undertreated.[5] Here I will describe the problem of pain at the end of life and then show a way to optimally manage pain in this vulnerable population.

The Problem: Pain and Its Pathophysiology

Pain, one of many forms of suffering, is common at the end of life and is usually accompanied by a plethora of other symptoms, including dyspnea, nausea, confusion, anxiety, and depression.[6] Pain seems to be the predominant symptom and also the most feared form of suffering.[7] Pain at the end of life is protean and complicated. No two patients are alike in terms of the pathophysiology of their pain complaints or the psychosocial contexts of their pain. Pain at the end of life is undertreated, which is completely preventable. There is an ethical obligation in medicine and nursing to relieve suffering, and it is this directive that should lead physicians and other providers, as well as society in general, to bring down barriers and optimize pain management throughout life, but particularly at the end of life.

The pathophysiology of pain is complex, with new scientific discoveries in this area occurring frequently. I will now explain the basic concepts of pain pathophysiology so as to inform the rationale for optimal pain-management strategies. *Nociception,* the most upstream signal in pain physiology, occurs when tissue damage results in the stimulation of peripheral neuroreceptors in tissues, which, in turn, transmit a signal to a peripheral nerve. *Transmission* is the traversing of a pain signal from the nociceptor to the peripheral nerve to the spinal cord to the brain stem to the midbrain to the sensory cortex to the association cortex. Next is *modulation,* when, at least at the levels from the spinal cord and above, descending and local signals serve to either dampen or accentuate the ascending pain signals from the periphery. After modulation comes *cognition,* the final, summed subjective sensation of pain and modifying influences as experienced by the patient. Finally, *expression* is the communication of this cognition to others, verbally or nonverbally. Although simplistic, this schema allows us to get from a painful site in the body to the point where the person suffering the pain tells the provider about the pain in the context of his or her life and illness, and also shows us the levels at which any intervention might have an impact upon the pain.

Assessment and Therapy

Thorough assessment of pain is absolutely vital in order to treat it optimally and manage the disease causing it appropriately. This is true for diseases in the end-of-life phase as well as eminently curable conditions. Important factors in the assessment of pain include determining the following: location—subjective and anatomic description of where the pain is situated; chronicity—the duration of the pain complaint; temporal pattern how the pain changes over time; severity—the intensity of the pain complaint, often measured from 0 to 10 (ordinal scale)[8] or on a visual analog scale;[9] character— how the pain is described, as sharp, dull, stabbing, burning, etc.; and associated findings at the end of life, many other findings may be present, including dyspnea, cachexia, fever, depression, etc. A comprehensive approach to treating pain, one that takes into account both its characteristics and the results of the workup indicating possible etiology and/or a unique pathophysiology, is most likely to be successful.

Assessment, workup, and therapy sometimes occur nearly simultaneously in the real-life situation, but in general, an initial assessment and treatment is usually followed as soon as possible by a thorough workup in the outpatient or inpatient setting. The workup includes a physical examination—a good general examination with special attention to the neurologic and musculoskeletal findings; laboratory examination—judicious use of laboratory tests to confirm or refute suspected conditions causing the pain complaint (for example, infection or bone metastasis); radiographic evaluation—targeted radiographs including plain films, computed tomography, ultrasound, magnetic resonance imaging, and even positron-emission tomography; and other tests—for example, biopsies would be required to confirm a diagnosis of primary cancer or recurrence, and pulmonary-function tests or echocardiogram would address the severity of chronic obstructive pulmonary disease or congestive heart failure at a given point in time. This evaluation narrows the possible causes of pain, which are usually still numerous in dying patients, and allows for targeted therapeutics.

Therapy should occur simultaneously with the workup process, not upon completion of the workup. Either the outpatient or inpatient setting may be appropriate for evaluation and management of pain, depending upon the severity of the symptoms and the ease of control. The primary physician, nurse, psychosocial professional, and consultants should be involved as indicated from the beginning and should have the ability to communicate on a daily and preferably in-person basis. Through the workup and therapy, the target of the efforts should be the pain experienced and described by the patient.

Physicians and nurses both tend to focus heavily on the pharmacologic management of pain, but it is important to point out that there are multiple other therapeutic modalities that can impact pain in a positive way, and that the right mix of modalities for a successful therapeutic plan will be different for each patient. In addition to pharmacologic agents, other modalities include surgical intervention, other interventional techniques, palliative or radical radiotherapy, physiatry, massage, and electromagnetic therapy (for example, ultrasound or electrical stimulation).

The principles of pharmacologic therapy for pain are well-established and have not changed dramatically in over three decades. Unfortunately, these principles are not being applied uniformly or effectively even in the United States. The World Health Organization formulated an analgesic-ladder concept in 1986 to serve as a guide to practitioners around the world regarding rational, effective use of non-opiate and opiate analgesics.[10] Opiates are the mainstay of pharmacologic therapy for pain at the end of life because they are safe, effective, and easy to use from a pharmacologic point of view. There is no maximum dose of any pure opiate agonist. These medications have several drawbacks, including regulatory constraints, limited supplies (in some countries), and the real but uncommon problems of abuse, diversion, and addiction. Opiates come in weak, moderate, and strong agents; single-agent versus combination products; long-acting versus short-acting formulations; and in forms for a variety of intended routes, including oral tablets/capsules, oral liquids, sublingual or transmucosal oral liquid or lozenge preparations, transdermal patches, suppositories, and solutions intended for the intravenous, subcutaneous, or intramuscular route. Most patients with chronic pain including at the end of life will do best with both a long-acting opiate formulation to prevent most pain and a short-acting opiate agent to treat episodic or breakthrough pain.[11] It is relatively simple to choose an appropriate agent(s), dose, route, and schedule, and most of the time, with follow-up and adjustment as needed, this plan of treatment will be successful. If not, switching to another type of opiate often works. This is called opiate rotation, and it is successful about 50 percent of the time.[12] In changing from one opiate agent to another, or from one route to another with the same or a different agent, an equianalgesic dosing table is quite helpful (see table 1.1).

Table 1.1. Equianalgesic Dosing Conversion Table

Oral or Rectal Dose (mg)	Agent	IV/IM/SQ Dose (mg)	Frequency
100	codeine	--	q 4-6h
15	hydrocodone	--	q 4-6h
10	oxycodone	--	q 4h
15	morphine	5	q 3-4h
4	hydromorphone	1.5	q 2-3h
--	fentanyl	25mcg/hr patch ~50mg morphine PO/24 hours	patch every 72h

Source: Adapted from Common physical symptoms. In: Emanuel LL, von Gunten CF, Hauser JM, eds. The Education in Palliative and End-of-Life Care (EPEC) Curriculum. Chicago: The EPEC Project; 1999, 2003.

In addition to opiates, other agents can have a direct or indirect effect on pain sensation or transmission. Traditionally, these other medications are called co-analgesics if they have analgesic properties on their own and adjuvant medications if they do not. The lines between these medications are becoming blurred as we learn more about their clinical and pharmacologic properties. Depending upon the type of pain—nociceptive, neuropathic, inflammatory, central, etc.—these other agents may add a great deal to what can be done with an opiate alone. In fact, on the WHO analgesic ladder, the first step is the use of acetaminophen or aspirin (or other nonsteroidal anti-inflammatory drugs [NSAIDs]) alone, without an opiate.[13] These weak analgesics can control mild pain, even at the end of life, in many patients. Other categories of adjuvants or co-analgesic medications include anti-inflammatory agents (corticosteroids and NSAIDs), true adjuvants/neuromodulators (tricyclic antidepressants, anticonvulsants), psychiatric agents (antidepressants, anxiolytics, neuroleptics), and topical agents (lidocaine lotion or patches, capsaicin cream). Other medications are commonly utilized to minimize side effects from opiates and similar medications; these include stool softeners, laxatives, antiemetics, antacid medications, psychostimulants, and sedatives.

Adequate control of pain at the end of life requires aggressive application of multimodality therapy as needed. Of course, the most simple and straightforward plan of care possible would be the preferred one, yet many patients at the end of life truly require multiple complementary medications and other therapies. The plan should be as aggressive and multifaceted as is needed to achieve the goal of reasonable comfort or minimal suffering, along with maximal cognitive and physical function, in the context of the underlying disease process. Rapid, frequent reassessment is vital. Reassessment includes serial pain-scale measurements over time, repeat physician visits with physical exams, appropriate laboratory tests and radiographs, nurse reassessments, and analysis of home health and hospice evaluations. Each assessment should be followed by appropriate alterations to the plan of care, along with updated education of the patient and family caregiver. Changes in old symptoms or the appearance of new ones warrants more thorough investigations to look for treatable etiologies of the new symptoms. Methods of controlling the side effects of the opiates and other effective medications should also be reassessed along the way and changed accordingly.

Conclusion

The problem of undertreated pain at the end of life is still a major challenge for health-care providers. In the United States, all of the resources to solve this problem are at hand. For the vast majority of patients, the full and judicious use of these resources will result in a satisfactory to excellent outcome in terms of control of pain and related symptoms. In only a small percentage of patients will refractory symptoms remain or interventional procedures be required. Still, financial, regulatory, and attitudinal constraints remain as the main impediments to reducing the burden of pain at the end of life. Disseminating knowledge and effecting change in attitudes and policies must accompany the increased application of modern pharmacologic and nonpharmacologic therapies in a multidisciplinary setting. Although new agents are on the horizon, their absence should not be an impediment to success in this arena today.

Notes

1. Von Roenn JH, Cleeland CS, Gonin R, et al. Physician attitudes and practice in cancer pain management: A survey from the Eastern Cooperative Oncology Group. *Ann Intern Med*. 1993;119:121–126.

2. World Health Organization. Cancer pain relief and palliative care. *Technical Report Series 804*. Geneva, Switzerland: World Health Organization; 1990.

3. American Academy of Pain Medicine and the American Pain Society. Consensus statement. *Clin J Pain*. 1997;13:68.

4. Ferrell BR, Ferrell BA. Pain in the elderly: A report of the task force on pain in the elderly of the International Association for the Study of Pain. Seattle: IASP Press; 1996.

5. Cleeland CS, Gonin R, Hatfield AK, et al. Pain and its treatment in outpatients with metastatic cancer. *NEJM*. 1994;330:592–596.

6. Curtis EB, Krech R, Walsh TD. Common symptoms in patients with advanced cancer. *J Palliat Care*. 1991;7:25–29.

7. Ng K, von Gunten CF. Symptoms and attitudes of 100 consecutive patients admitted to an acute hospice/palliative care unit. *J Pain Symptom Manage*. 1998;16:307–316.

8. Jensen MP, Karoly P, Braver S. The measurement of clinical pain intensity: A comparison of six methods. *Pain*. 1986;27:117–126.

9. Ferraz MB, Quaresma MR, Aquino LR, et al. Reliability of pain scales in the assessment of literate and illiterate patients with rheumatoid arthritis. *J Rheumatol*. 1990;17:1022–1024.

10. World Health Organization. *Cancer Pain Relief*. Geneva, Switzerland: World Health Organization; 1986.

11. Portnoy RK, Hagen NA. Breakthrough pain: Definition, prevalence, and characteristics. *Pain*. 1990;41:273–281.

12. Watanabe S. Intraindividual variability in opioid response: A role for sequential opioid trials in patient care. In: Portnoy RK, Bruera E, eds. *Topics in Palliative Care*, vol. 1. New York: Oxford University Press; 1997:195–203.

13. World Health Organization. *Cancer Pain Relief*. Geneva, Switzerland: World Health Organization; 1986.

2
Relieving Pain: Today's Legal and Ethical Risks
David A. Fleming

In June 2001, a California jury found an internist liable for reckless neglect in undertreating a dying man's pain and ordered the physician to pay $1.5 million to his patient's surviving family members.[1] The finding of negligence in this case was not due to improper diagnosis or treatment of a disease, but was based solely on inadequate pain control. This landmark case marked the first time a jury had determined that physician neglect constituted elder abuse. The physician's argument in this case was that more aggressive treatment with narcotics would have hastened the patient's death by depressing respiration. His fear was that causing the death of the patient in this way would have placed him at risk for civil action, or could have led to disciplinary action or even criminal charges. This case has set a legal precedent. While physicians in this country historically have worried that they could face criminal prosecution or regulatory action for overprescribing controlled substances, this verdict warns that underprescribing may be just as risky legally. As observed by a representative of the Compassion in Dying Federation, "Failure to treat pain is something that physicians can now be held accountable for."[2]

When facing the complexities of care at the end of life, everyone—patient, nurse, physician, and caregiver alike—endorses the importance of providing adequate relief from pain and suffering.[3] This attitude of compassion and caring is the grounding principle of the healing profession. Yet health-care providers in this country still do not do a good enough job of relieving pain, even when the most up-to-date advancements in medical technology and drugs are available. Patients with terminal illnesses often fear pain and suffering more than death itself, which is why many express a desire to end life well before the indignity of suffering is upon them.[4] Such fears are well founded. Between 10 and 50 percent of patients in programs devoted to palliative care report significant pain shortly before death.[5] Investigators in an extensive nationwide study of end-of-life care found that even after an intervention designed to inform physicians about patient preferences and improve palliative care, there was no improvement in either pain control or other aspects of treatment for terminally ill patients.[6]

The barriers to adequate palliative care are substantial. Society as a whole, and subsequently its health-care providers, tends to view the subject of death as anathema to good health care. Death is the enemy; it must be "defeated," not acquiesced to. Other barriers that frequently limit good palliative care are time limitations in busy medical practices and prognostic uncertainty by the health-care team as the patient deteriorates. More often, however, the barriers to aggressive pain control are fear of reprisal, a poor understanding about the use of narcotic drugs and addiction, avoidance of the subject, and otherwise inadequate communication between the patient and the provider.[7]

Physicians understand the obligations of their profession and the oath that they took to help suffering people.[8] However, end-of-life issues historically have not been emphasized in training, and physicians are often ill equipped to meet the challenge of palliative care. Physicians tend to fear reprisal if they are viewed as "giving up" too soon or as prescribing narcotics too heavily. There also may be unavoidable conflict between the expectations of the patient and family, who want pain medication, and the judgment of the physician, who fears professional sanction or penalties from the Drug Enforcement Agency (DEA) when individual prescribing practices are scrutinized. Increasing awareness of this concern has encouraged research and generated numerous published articles underscoring the need for greater understanding of the ethics and laws governing the use of opioids and other controlled substances, as well as better pain-management skills in physicians.

Increasingly, medical societies, academic think tanks, health-care organizations, public-health groups, consumer groups, and state and federal governments are identifying pain management as a priority, especially for patients with chronic illness who are dying. In a recent report by the Institute of Medicine, *Approaching Death: Improving Care at the End-of-life*, there was a call to action at all levels to accept death as a part of life, to improve care at the end of life, and to assure people that they will be neither abandoned nor maltreated as they approach death.[9] The expectation of cure at all costs, professional regulation, and fears of litigation have created barriers in clinical practice and in professional training. But there is now an unprecedented trend to create good policy in order to appropriately regulate medical practice and the use of controlled substances without jeopardizing patient welfare.

The Changing Legal Environment

The federal government has attempted to regulate potentially addictive and harmful medications for almost one hundred years. With growing concern about the control and distribution of opioids in this country, and the illegal use and wide availability of narcotics in the 1960s, the United States Congress in 1970 passed the Controlled Substances Act (CSA), which acknowledges the legitimacy of prescribing narcotics and hypnotics, but monitors and regulates their use.[10] The CSA goes further to confirm that physicians have an obligation to "first do no harm" and to treat patients who are suffering from intractable pain. To meet the needs of the elderly and disabled who are terminally ill, Congress provided for Medicare hospice benefits in the Tax Equity and Fiscal Responsibility Act of 1984. To confirm patients' rights to refuse treatment, Congress also passed the Uniform Rights for the Terminally Ill Act in 1989 and the Patient Self-determination Act in 1990. Both of these laws protect patients' right of refusal, but not their right to adequate palliative care or assisted death in the face of terminal illness.

With growing concern over misuse of prescription drugs and the administration of lethal overdoses to dying patients, Congress amended the CSA in 1984, empowering the DEA to revoke physicians' federal drug licenses if they used controlled substances to "endanger health and safety," regardless of whether state law was violated.[11] The status of the DEA had shifted from being a monitoring security agency to being a policing regulatory agency with the power to severely sanction practicing physicians if they were substantively "out of scope" of practice standards. The agency's ability to sanction has had a chilling effect on the willingness of many physicians to prescribe narcotics, even when indicated.

State policies regarding the use of controlled substances may be more restrictive than those of the federal government. Many state laws do not recognize the value of using narcotics or that their use is standard medical practice. Some states' statutes perpetuate the belief that opioids unduly hasten death.[12] In other states, however, pain-treatment statutes specifically identify the use of opioids and pain management as being part of medical practice and encourage appropriate prescribing. In Missouri, for instance, the controlled-substances statute restricts narcotic prescriptions to a thirty-day supply, but the supply may be increased to up to three months if the physician describes on the prescription the medical indications for a larger supply.[13] The Missouri law also explicitly states that "no physician shall be subject to disciplinary action by the board solely for prescribing, administering or dispensing controlled substances when prescribed, administered or dispensed for the therapeutic purpose for a person diagnosed and treated by a physician for a condition resulting in intractable pain, if such diagnosis and treatment has been documented in the physician's medical records." The key word is *documented*. As in every aspect of medical practice, physicians should maintain good documentation to support their prescribing habits.

Current federal law, most state laws, and DEA regulations acknowledge that prescribing opioids is appropriate for the treatment of pain, and that there is no intent to limit physicians' prescribing for intractable pain, even if the use of such substances may increase the risk of death.[14] The United States Supreme Court has also recognized that patients suffering from terminal illness have a constitutional right to adequate palliative care even if such treatment hastens death.[15] The Supreme Court stops short, however, of recognizing a patient's "right" to assisted death. The recent statutory trend has been toward improving the knowledge and skill of providers, and encouraging the appropriate use of opioids for intractable pain. Over the past few years, however, several legislative agendas have once again cast fear and doubt on the aggressive use of these medications for pain relief.

In 1995, Oregon became the first state government to allow physicians to prescribe controlled substances to assist the suicide of patients with terminal illness and intractable pain who have requested help to die.[16] Oregon law allows physicians to legally act in direct violation of the Controlled Substances Act of 1970. Recognizing Oregon's right to govern itself, then United States Attorney General Janet Reno created an exception to the CSA in 1998 indicating that no adverse action would be taken against Oregon physicians who were in compliance with state law. This sequence of events brought strong reaction on both sides of the argument regarding physician-assisted death.[17]

In response, members of the United States Congress introduced the Legal Drug Abuse Prevention Act in 1998 with the goal of overriding Reno's decision and halting Oregon's legalization of physician-assisted suicide. This bill, which became the Pain Relief Promotion Act of 1999, was met with resistance from the American Medical Association (AMA) and other proponents of palliative care who were fearful of the chilling effect that such a law would have on physicians and their willingness to aggressively treat pain.[18] Ultimately, the "Pain Bill" was modified to incorporate phrasing that strongly encouraged appropriate standards of palliative care, which then garnered support from the AMA and hospice organizations, but the strong punitive components remained, including threats of imprisonment, fines, and loss of licensure. Resistance to the punitive aspects of this bill has continued from patients and physicians, who are fearful that patients will suffer for want of pain relief because cautious physicians may hold back when prescribing narcotics.[19]

The Pain Relief Promotion Act remained dormant, for the most part due to the actions of then United States Attorney General John Ashcroft, until November 2001, when Ashcroft removed the Reno exception for Oregon physicians and instructed DEA agents to move against those who used controlled substances in violation of the Controlled Substances Act of 1970.[20] The order did not call for criminal prosecution of doctors, but did permit suspension and revocation of drug licenses. In support of palliative care, the Ashcroft order did stipulate that pain management was a valid medical use of controlled substances.

The legal environment of the medical practice of relieving pain remains in flux at both the state and the federal level. State statutes may conflict with federal law, and both are susceptible to interpretation. In general, professional societies, government organizations, and state boards tend to encourage the use of narcotics for pain relief, but the prescribing habits of physicians are still under scrutiny. In today's medical-legal environment, the threat of retribution and litigation continues to forestall many physicians' prescribing practices and subsequently to limit the effectiveness of palliative care.

Ethical Conflicts When Treating Pain

The ethical norms guiding treatment of suffering patients are incontestable. Physicians, quite simply, have an obligation to do everything in their power to relieve pain and suffering because that is what they are supposed to do as physicians. The obligation to serve the patient's welfare is met not only by doing what is best for the patient clinically, but also by having compassion, integrity, and respect for the values, beliefs, and wishes of the patient. Every activity of medicine should be guided by the beneficence of the caregiver and the trust cultivated in the relationship that is formed between patients and their health-care providers.[21] The principle of beneficence obligates health care professionals to ease the burden of suffering during the natural course of disease and death. This duty requires efforts to alleviate both physical and emotional suffering through appropriate means, as established by professional standards and the laws of society.

These claims are impressive, even imposing, and can be very useful when doing an ethical analysis of a clinical situation or when making an intellectual argument. But for the clinician who deals with the day-to-day intricacies of illness and death, there are many competing issues that pertain and that should be factored into the ethical calculation. Clinical circumstances can be unclear, and the use of analgesics is often minimized until diagnostic accuracy is established. Also, physicians typically want to remain in good standing with their colleagues, the DEA, and their state licensing boards, all of which have review processes, along with laws, regulations, and by-laws that may be unclear or difficult to interpret. These professional concerns are legitimate. Finally, many physicians have strongly held beliefs regarding the use of drugs that can hasten death, and the values and beliefs of physicians also deserve respect. The welfare of physicians is a concern because, in addition to the dying patient, there are many other patients for whom the integrity and sustainability of their physician is important.

These arguments for consideration of the physician's interests are compelling, but what is the patient's view from the gurney? The patient and the physician exist in a covenantal relationship that consists of one simple understanding: physicians promise to be there for patients, who, in turn, trust that physicians will keep that promise. This is not to say that physicians and nurses must, or even can, be physically at the patient's side continuously, but we can provide the assurance that we will use our knowledge and skill, and that care will be delivered in a coordinated fashion by a skilled team of providers. Incorporated in this pledge is the promise that patients will not be slighted at their time of greatest need. This is a challenging expectation in modern health-care systems. Patient care, especially palliative care, requires a delicate balancing of needs with responses, which encompass more than the isolated application of principles, personal belief, medical science, or the laws of society. It requires all of that with the singular goal of helping the patient.

Today's physicians no longer have the luxury of being the sole proprietors of health-care decisions. Many interested parties now lay claim to the decisions that direct the care of patients. These parties move together in a complex matrix of accountability, and they share responsibility for the outcome.[22] Integrated health-care systems, insurance plans, employers, government regulators, state boards, medical staffs, and provider groups all participate as stakeholders in the "insured lives" of patients. The physician, as one of many "interested parties," is often linked to others through independent contracts that demand accountability independent of the patient.

These outside contracts ethically obligate physicians, but only to the extent that they are capable of providing the needed services contracted for and that in doing so they need not abdicate strongly held moral beliefs or jeopardize the welfare of their patients. From an ethical as well as legal standpoint this means that physicians should document well and communicate effectively with patients and other members of the health-care team. A typical requirement of most physicians' contracts is that they sustain the knowledge and skill necessary for their assigned duties or provide appropriate referral to another physician when necessary. As members of society, physicians are obligated to follow the laws of society, but they must also be ready and willing to advocate for improvements in health policy when necessary.

When using narcotics in the treatment of terminally ill patients, the rule of double effect can be applied if the patient is unduly suffering and beyond hope of cure, and if the intent is to relieve suffering. The ethical argument is that there is good intent in attempting to relieve the patient's suffering, even knowing that death may be hastened as a consequence of giving narcotics or other drugs that tend to suppress respiration with higher dosing.[23] This premise is well established and accepted both ethically and legally, but many physicians are hesitant to apply this doctrine because of personal belief that they will be "overdosing" the patient, even when the patient is suffering terribly with terminal illness. It can also be troublesome when the patient's clinical situation or prognosis is unclear or when there is still some hope for clinical improvement, which may then heighten concern about accelerating death. Establishing intent is crucial, both legally and ethically. The intention and expectation of the health-care team, as well as the expectation of the patient, should be well documented in the medical record;

such documentation also provides a reference point for further decision making as the clinical circumstances evolve.

Conclusion

Pain and other forms of discomfort are prominent contributors to physical suffering in patients with terminal illness, but these symptoms tend to be undertreated. The enlightenment provided by clinical research and training holds out hope that there will be better understanding of suffering and the development of new, more effective palliative treatments.[24] It is important that physicians keep their attitudes, knowledge, and understanding about care at the end of life up to date, with awareness of the legal environment and the commonly agreed-upon ethical precepts that inform palliative care.

Federal and state agencies recognize that controlled substances, including opioids, are often essential in the treatment of acute and chronic pain. Model guidelines explicitly state that physicians should not fear disciplinary action from regulatory boards or enforcement agencies when prescribing, dispensing, or administering controlled substances, including opioid analgesics, for legitimate medical purposes.[25]

The legal environment in this country continues to offer mixed messages, but it appears to be moving toward encouraging better-trained physicians who know how to use controlled substances appropriately and will use them aggressively when needed. This is not to say that regulation and scrutiny of prescribing practices will cease to occur, nor does it discount the need for good documentation. These requirements will continue as a natural part of regulation.

The ethical dimensions of pain relief for dying patients are complicated and at times difficult to navigate, and they will always challenge the thoughtful physician who considers the primacy of patient welfare in the context of other legitimate obligations. Remaining knowledgeable in the science of medicine and in the laws that pertain will strengthen physicians' ability to act without fear. Above all, physicians must take the time to document well and to communicate effectively with patients, their families, and other members of the health-care team in order to gain a clear understanding of the goals and values informing end-of-life decisions.

Notes

1. Okie S. California jury finds doctor negligent in managing pain. *Washington Post.* June 15, 2001:A2.

2. Crane M. Treating pain: Damned if you don't. *Medical Economics.* November 19, 2001:66–68.

3. Steinhauser KE, Christakis NA, Clipp ED, et al. Factors considered important at the end-of-life by patients, family, physicians, and other care providers. *JAMA.* 2000;284(19):2476–2482.

4. Quill T. Death with dignity: A case of individualized decision-making. *NEJM.* 1991;324:691–694.

5. Quill T. Palliative options of last resort: A comparison of voluntary stopping of eating and drinking, terminal sedation, physician-assisted suicide and voluntary euthanasia. *JAMA.* 1995;278(23):2099–2104.

6. The SUPPORT Principal Investigators. A controlled trial to improve care for seriously ill hospitalized patients: The Study to Understand Prognosis and Preferences for Outcomes and Risks of Treatments (SUPPORT). *JAMA.* 1995;274(20):1591–1598.

7. Byock I, Caplan A, Snyder L. Beyond symptom management: Physician roles and responsibility in palliative care. In: Snyder L, Quill T, eds. *Physician's Guide to End-of-Life Care.* Philadelphia: American College of Physicians; 2001:56–71.

8. American College of Physicians. Ethics manual. 4th ed. *Ann Intern Med.* 1998;128:576–594. Oath of Hippocrates. In: Etziony M. *The Physician's Creed: An Anthology of Medical Prayers, Oaths, and Codes of Ethics Written and Recited by Medical Practitioners through the Ages.* Springfield, IL: Charles C. Thomas; 1973:13–14.

9. Institute of Medicine. *Approaching Death: Improving Care at the End-of-life.* Washington, DC: National Academy Press; 1997.

10. Code of Federal Regulations, Title 21, pt. 1306.04a, www.deadivision.usdoj.gov/21CFR/806 (accessed 10/24/09).

11. Code of Federal Regulations, Title 21, United States Code, Controlled Substances Act, www.deadivision.usdoj.gov/21CFR/21USC/802 (accessed 10–24–09).

12. Pain and Policy Studies Group. *Achieving Balance in Federal and State Pain Policy.* 2000. http://www.painpolicy.wisc.edu (accessed 10–23–09).

13. *Uniform Controlled Substances Act.* 195.101 R.S. MO.

14. *DEA Physician's Manual.* Washington, DC: Government Printing Office; March 1990:21.

15. *Glucksberg v. Washington,* 117 S. Ct. 2258 (1997); *Quill v. Vacco,* 117 S. Ct. 2293 (1997).

16. Oregon Death with Dignity Act, ballot measure no. 16 (November 8, 1994): Revised Statute 127.800–995 (1995).

17. Kill the pain, not the patient (editorial). *The Oregonian.* July 1, 1999; Annas G. Death by prescription—the Oregon initiative. *NEJM.* 1994; 331(18):1240–1243.

18. Orentlicher D, Caplan A. The Pain Relief Promotion Act of 1999: A serious threat to palliative care. *JAMA.* 2000;283(2):255–258.

19. Walsh, B. Side effect of suicide bill criticized. *Times Picayune* (New Orleans, LA). September 21, 2000.

20. Ashcroft allows agents to go after suicide assistance. *USA Today.* November 6, 2001. http://www.usatoday.com/news/washdc/nov01/2001-11-06-ashcroft.htm.

21. Pellegrino E, Thomasma DC. *For the Good of the Patient: The Restoration of Beneficence in Health Care.* New York: Oxford University Press; 1988:51–58.

22. Emanuel E, Emanuel L. What is accountability in health care? *Ann Intern Med.* 1996;124:229–239.

23. Beauchamp TL, Childress JF. *Principles of Biomedical Ethics.* 5th ed. New York: Oxford University Press; 2001:128–132.

24. Management of cancer symptoms: Pain, depression, and fatigue. Evidence Report/Technology Assessment: Number 61. Agency for Healthcare Research and Quality pub. no. 02-E061. 2002. http://www.ahrq.gov/clinic/epcsums/csympsum.htm.

25. Missouri Board of Healing Arts. Model guidelines for the use of controlled substances for the treatment of pain. *Healing Arts News.* 2002;(Spring)17(1):4–7.

3
Relieving Non-pain Suffering at the End of Life
Clay M. Anderson

The term *disease* implies both a pathologic biological process in a person and a burden of suffering upon the person. It is considered an obligation of the compassionate physician and health-care team not only to treat disease, but also to manage symptoms in order to minimize suffering and maximize comfort throughout the disease trajectory. At the end of life, when disease-modifying treatments are no longer available, not advisable, or not desired by the patient, care becomes focused on the whole person and treatment becomes focused on symptom management—often discontinuing consideration for the cause of the symptoms. The overall care of a patient, focused on the whole person and his or her values and goals, is just as important as specific symptom-focused interventions. Symptoms can be caused by the underlying chronic-disease process, other associated diseases or conditions, prior treatment, and psychological/emotional factors. Treatments are directed at the pathophysiology of the symptom, and so are usually the same regardless of the underlying disease.

A person near the end of life may develop many problematic symptoms. Here I will discuss the evaluation and management of dyspnea, nausea and vomiting, constipation, diarrhea, bowel obstruction, anorexia, fatigue/weakness, edema, skin ulcers, and insomnia. It is worth noting that people fear pain the most, but they also fear these other symptoms, as well as loss of control and dignity.[1]

While pain management is often foremost in the minds of physicians providing end-of-life care, the above-mentioned symptoms can be as distressing as pain to patients and their caregivers. The basic approach to evaluating a symptom is the same as that used to manage an illness: taking an accurate history, performing a thorough physical examination, and running appropriate laboratory or imaging investigations. Often goals of care may preclude disease management, or the patient may be in the last hours of life, when arranging imaging studies or awaiting laboratory investigations is simply not appropriate. It is important to become confident and competent at "treating without diagnosing" in these circumstances. Initiating therapeutic trials based on inference and monitoring patients' responses can provide both symptom relief for patients and additional information regarding symptom pathophysiology for physicians.

Dyspnea

Dyspnea may be caused by anemia, airway obstruction, anxiety, bronchospasm, hypoxemia, pleural effusion, pneumonia, pulmonary edema, pulmonary embolism, metabolic disturbances, or emotional and environmental insults.[2] If pneumonia is suspected, it should be treated in a manner consistent with the patient's wishes, including the use of antibiotics and antipyretics, as appropriate. Often it will not be possible to determine or correct the underlying cause. Medical management of this symptom consists of using oxygen, opiates, and anxiolytics. Nonpharmacologic measures, such as body and bed positioning, can greatly ease the suffering of breathlessness.

It is important to note that most patients who report breathlessness are not hypoxemic.[3] Pulse oximetry is not as reliable or helpful as is the patient's self-report. Cool air moving across a patient's face may eliminate dyspnea as effectively as supplemental oxygen will. However, a trial of supplemental oxygen may be beneficial, and since most patients consider oxygen supplementation to be the standard modern treatment for dyspnea, they may expect it.

Opiates relieve breathlessness in many patients, possibly by both central and peripheral mechanisms. Doses lower than those required to achieve pain control are often successful. While anecdotal reports abound maintaining that nebulized opiates are effective, they have not been shown to have advantages over oral or parenteral regimens.[4] When dosing guidelines are followed, respiratory depression, hastened death, or abusive behaviors are not likely.

Opiates alone do not reliably relieve anxiety in many breathless patients, and since breathlessness is often associated with anxiety and vice versa, some dyspneic patients may require additional treatment focused on anxiety. Benzodiazepines are effective, preferably using relatively longer half-life preparations to avoid pronounced peak/trough effects. They are safe to use in conjunction with opiates. See table 3.1 for suggested doses of some benzodiazepines.

Table 3.1. Benzodiazepines for Dyspnea

MEDICATION	DOSE	ROUTE OF ADMINISTRATION	FREQUENCY
lorazepam	0.5-2.0 mg	PO, SL, or IV	q 1h until effect, then q 4-6h
diazepam	5-10 mg	PO or IV	q 1h until effect, then q 6-8h
clonazepam	0.25-2.0 mg	PO	q 12h
midazolam	0.5 mg	IV	q 15min until effect, then continuous SQ or IV

Source: Adapted from Common physical symptoms. In: Emanuel LL, von Gunten CF, Hauser JM, eds. The Education in Palliative and End-of-Life Care (EPEC) Curriculum. Chicago: The EPEC Project; 1999, 2003.

Patients with audible wheezing or other signs of bronchoconstriction, or those who are known or suspected to have reactive airways due to asthma or chronic obstructive pulmonary disease, should have a trial of adrenergic or anticholinergic bronchodilators by nebulizer, metered-dose inhaler, or both. A lack of subjective benefit after an adequate trial should usually lead to termination of this strategy, which can interfere with other beneficial interventions. Cough suppressants, expectorants, mucolytics, and adequate hydration are also worth trying in many patients.

Nonpharmacologic measures may be beneficial in relieving dyspnea and can be effective alone. A cool but comfortable room is ideal, with adequate humidity and free of environmental irritants such as smoke. A window is desirable, open, if possible, with an unobstructed view to the outside. Only a limited number of people should be allowed in the room to avoid crowding. Relaxation, distraction, or hypnotic therapy may also be beneficial. Body and bed positioning to gain mechanical advantage and principles of pulmonary toilet will also often yield positive results.

Nausea and Vomiting

Nausea is a subjective sensation related to cortical responses or stimulation of the gastrointestinal lining, the chemoreceptor trigger zone in the brain, or the vestibular apparatus. Neurotransmitters involved in this include serotonin, dopamine, acetylcholine, and histamine. Cortical responses, such as anticipatory nausea associated with chemotherapy, seem to be learned and are not associated with specific neurotransmitters. The causes of nausea and vomiting can be thought of as the "Eleven Ms": metastases, meningeal irritation, movement, mental anxiety, medications, mucosal irritation, mechanical obstruction, motility, metabolic disruption, microbes, and myocardial weakness.[5]

Different causes will require different measures for ideal control of nausea. Medications that can be helpful include the following: antacids, anticholinergics, antihistamines, cytoprotective agents, dopamine antagonists, prokinetic agents, and serotonin antagonists. The most common form of nausea is probably dopamine mediated. Haloperidol is the least sedating dopamine antagonist. See table 3.2 for recommended doses of dopamine antagonists for treating dopamine-mediated nausea. Antihistamines that also have anticholinergic activity may be beneficial. Examples are diphenhydramine, meclizine, and hydroxyzine. Doses of 25–50 mg PO q 6h are usually effective.

MEDICATION	DOSE	ROUTE OF ADMINISTRATION	FREQUENCY
haloperidol	0.5-2.0 mg	PO, IV, or SC	q 6h, then titrate
prochlorperazine	10-20 mg	PO or PR	q 6h, q 12h respectively
prochlorperazine	5-10 mg	IV	q 6h
droperidol	2.5-5.0 mg	IV	q 6h
promethazine	12.5-25 mg	PO, PR, or IV	q 4-6h
metoclopramide	10-20 mg	PO	q 6h

Table 3.2. Dopamine Antagonists for Nausea and Vomiting

Source: Adapted from Common physical symptoms. In: Emanuel LL, von Gunten CF, Hauser JM, eds. The Education in Palliative and End-of-Life Care (EPEC) Curriculum. Chicago: The EPEC Project; 1999, 2003.

Anticholinergics can diminish opiate- or anesthetic-related nausea that is acetylcholine mediated via the vestibular apparatus. One could consider using scopolamine; suggested doses are 0.1–0.4 mg SC or IV q 4h, or 1–3 transdermal patches (1.5 mg) q 72h, or 10–80 mcg/h continuous IV or SC infusion.

Serotonin antagonists can be very effective but are quite expensive. They are usually tried only when other medications have failed. Medications that can be tried include the following: ondansetron 8 mg PO tid or granisetron 1 mg PO qd or bid.

Prokinetic agents may be beneficial for nausea related to the sluggish bowel of carcinomatosis, opiate therapy, or use of other medications, or to pseudo-obstruction from a large liver, ascites, or peritoneal disease. The medication most commonly used is metaclopramide 10–20 mg PO q 6h (before meals and at bedtime).

Nausea related to hyperacidity, esophageal reflux, or gastric or duodenal ulceration/erosions may be treated with 15–30 cc of antacid q 2h PRN; histamine-2-receptor antagonists such as cimetidine, ranitidine, or famotidine; or proton-pump inhibitors such as omeprazole, lansoprazole, or esomeprazole.

Other medications that have unclear mechanisms of action but evidence and experience of benefit in some patients include the following: dexamethasone 6–20 mg PO qd, dronabinol 2.5–5 mg PO tid, or lorazepam 0.5–2.0 mg PO q 4–6h.

Constipation

Constipation may be caused by medications, decreased motility, ileus, mechanical obstruction, dehydration, metabolic abnormalities, spinal-cord compression, autonomic dysfunction, or malignancy.[6] Unmanaged constipation leads to suffering from abdominal pain, bloating, nausea and vomiting, overflow incontinence, tenesmus, fecal impaction, or bowel obstruction. General measures that can be helpful include regular toileting based on the patient's normal bowel pattern and exploiting the gastrocolic reflex that occurs after eating.

Stimulant laxatives, usually combined with the stool softener docusate sodium, work by irritating the bowel and increasing peristalsis, and they are usually helpful. These agents should always be initiated when opiate therapy is begun in order to prevent inevitable opiate-associated constipation. Prevention of severe constipation is much preferable to treating the problem once it is manifest. Stimulant laxatives should be administered routinely and escalated as needed.

Cathartics may be required in constipated patients with advanced disease, poor mobility, and diminished oral intake. Osmotic agents draw water into the bowel lumen, maintaining or increasing the moisture content and overall volume of stool. Stool softeners, used alone for mild constipation, are detergent laxatives that facilitate the dissolution of fat in water and increase the water content of stool. Lubricant stimulants both lubricate the stool and irritate the bowel, creating increased peristalsis. Examples are glycerin suppositories and mineral or peanut oil. Large-volume enemas add water to stool and distend the bowel, inducing peristalsis. Soap suds added to a water enema create more bowel irritation, stimulating additional peristalsis. See table 3.3 for listings of some of these agents.

Table 3.3. Treatments for Constipation			
AGENT	DOSE	ROUTE OF ADMINISTRATION	FREQUENCY
STIMULANT LAXATIVES			
prune juice	120-240 cc	PO	qd or bid
senna	2 tablets	PO -- titrate to effect (9 or more per day)	q hs
casanthranol	2 tablets	PO -- titrate to effect (9 or more per day)	q hs
bisacodyl	5 mg	PO or PR -- titrate to effect	q hs
OSMOTIC AGENTS			
lactulose	30 cc initially	PO -- titrate to effect	q 4-6h
sorbitol 70%	30 cc initially	PO -- titrate to effect	q 4-6h
polyethylene glycol	17 g initially	in juice or water PO then titrate to effect	qd to bid
magnesium citrate	1-2 bottles	PO	PRN
STOOL SOFTENERS			
sodium docusate	1-2 tablets	PO -- titrate to effect	qd to bid
calcium docusate	1-2 tablets	PO -- titrate to effect	qd to bid
phosphosoda	enema	PR	qd

Source: Adapted from Common physical symptoms. In: Emanuel LL, von Gunten CF, Hauser JM, eds. The Education in Palliative and End-of-Life Care (EPEC) Curriculum. Chicago: The EPEC Project; 1999, 2003.

Diarrhea

Infections, gastrointestinal bleeding, malabsorption, medications, obstruction, overflow incontinence, stress, or lack of absorptive surface may cause diarrhea.[7] Keys to conservative management involve establishing what is normal for the patient and then making dietary adjustments to eliminate gas-producing foods and to increase bulk. Pharmacologic therapy is required when diarrhea is moderate to severe or has become chronic.

Mild or transient diarrhea can be managed with attapulgite (for example, Kaopectate) 30 cc or 2 tablets PRN, or bismuth salts (for example, Pepto-Bismol) 15–30 cc bid–qid. Persistent diarrhea is best managed with agents that slow peristalsis, including opiates. Treatment options are listed in table 3.4. Severe, secretory diarrhea may be managed with octreotide 50 mcg SC q 8–12h; titrate to 500 mcg or higher q 8h. Provide parenteral fluid support if necessary and appropriate.

MEDICATION	DOSE	ROUTE OF ADMINISTRATION	FREQUENCY
loperamide	2-4 mg	PO	q 6h or higher
diphenoxalate	2.5-5.0 mg	PO	q 6h or higher
tincture of opium	0.7 cc	PO	q 4h and titrate
MS Contin	15 mg	PO	bid
octreotide	100-500 mcg	SQ	q 8h

Table 3.4. Treatments for Diarrhea

Source: Adapted from Common physical symptoms. In: Emanuel LL, von Gunten CF, Hauser JM, eds. The Education in Palliative and End-of-Life Care (EPEC) Curriculum. Chicago: The EPEC Project; 1999, 2003.

Bowel Obstruction

Bowel obstruction, usually from metastatic cancer, causes nausea, vomiting, belching, distention, abdominal cramping, abdominal pain, constipation, and diarrhea. This can be a major challenge for the dying patient, and is quite difficult to manage medically. Mechanical interventions include surgical bypass or resection, gastrostomy, or nasogastric tube drainage.[8] While these interventions may be appropriate in incurable patients early in the course of their illnesses, their appropriateness declines over time as harms begin to outweigh benefits. Bowel obstruction can be managed medically, and it usually requires aggressive intervention and frequent reassessment. Bowel rest (no oral intake) is not required, but will usually help, even if it is only partial. The patient will usually have to be sedated to a greater or lesser degree to achieve adequate relief from bowel obstruction. A balanced approach using opiates, antispasmodics, benzodiazepines, and antipsychotics is most effective.[9] Corticosteroids may also treat any inflammatory component, if suspected. Rectal, subcutaneous, or intravenous routes of administration are often required. Obstruction may remit spontaneously for a time, allowing temporary removal of medications, an improved level of alertness, and perhaps resumption of some oral intake for enjoyment's sake.

Anorexia

Loss of appetite and loss of weight are commonly encountered in the end stages of many diseases. Caregivers and even patients often mistakenly believe they must be doing something wrong in these circumstances. It is important to provide education that these symptoms usually represent the natural progression of disease and are not reversible. It is reasonable, however, to search for potentially correctable problems that may be adding to the patient's suffering (for example, dysphagia, odynophagia, medication effects, or infections).

Although therapies that improve appetite or stimulate weight gain do not add to longevity, patients and caregivers will usually appreciate the semblance of normalcy associated with eating for enjoyment. Still, the patient who is not hungry should not be coerced into eating for any reason, since enjoyment of the food is the primary goal and cannot be achieved by force. Beneficial measures include the following: 1) eliminate any dietary restrictions, 2) offer favorite foods, and supplements if desired, 3) suggest an alcoholic beverage such as a glass of wine, and 4) administer dexamethasone 2–20 mg PO qd; megestrol acetate 200 mg PO q 6–8h and titrate; dronabinol (Marinol)—begin with small doses and titrate to effect; or androgens (oxandrolone, nandrolone).

Fatigue/Weakness

Fatigue/weakness is frequently listed as one of the most bothersome symptoms for patients with advanced illness. Management begins with helping patients and caregivers learn to alter activities to promote energy conservation. Transfusion for anemia-associated fatigue early on in the course of illness can be beneficial. Treating anemia with erythropoietin agents, which are not usually useful at the end of life due to delayed effect and expense, is falling out of favor due to emerging data showing uncommon but real toxicities and risks. Physical therapists and occupational therapists can help evaluate the situation, educate the patient and caregivers in energy conservation, and provide appropriate assistive devices. Stopping routine medications that are being taken for chronic illness but may no longer be appropriate at the end of life may help diminish fatigue. This is one area where physical assistance (for example, two caregivers assisting a person to his or her garden or using a wheelchair for a short day trip to a favorite outdoor spot) can allow patients to achieve their goals without making the symptom better.

Few medications are beneficial in treating fatigue/weakness at the end of life, but steroids and/or psychostimulants may be beneficial. The following are possible treatments and suggested doses: 1) dexamethasone 2–20 mg PO qd; 2) methylphenidate 2.5–5 mg PO q am and q noon, titrate to 10–30 mg/dose; 3) pemoline 25–100 mg bid; 4) dextroamphetamine 5 mg q am and q noon, titrate to 10–20 mg/dose.

Edema

Edema that has an easily identifiable and reversible cause should be treated appropriately. Judicious use of diuretics is reasonable. That being said, patients with advanced disease and hypoalbuminemia will be unable to maintain normal intravascular volume. Albumin infusions are inappropriate; they are expensive, ineffective, and frequently exacerbate problems with edema. A small amount of edema is expected in patients with hypoalbuminemia—lack of edema usually signifies significant dehydration in this setting. Patients and caregivers should be reassured that urine output of 300 cc/d or less is adequate. Patients should be encouraged to eat and drink as they normally would, but supplemental fluids should be avoided. Some salt-containing fluids (for example, soups, sports drinks, vegetable juices) should be encouraged in place of free water drinks such as water, tea, coffee, and soft drinks.

Caregivers should maximize comfort by paying careful attention to keeping mucous membranes moist and well lubricated (lips, mouth, eyes, nose). It is common for patients in the last hours of life to lose thirst, and family and caregivers should be educated regarding this change. Providing unwanted fluids could increase secretions that may further impair breathing, add to misery from incontinence in debilitated patients, and worsen edema states.

Some patients may be more comfortable with compression bandages applied to edematous limbs. Leg elevation and/or compression stockings are other options.

Skin Ulcers

Skin ulcers are more easily prevented than treated. Family members and caregivers should be instructed regarding the importance of keeping the patient's skin clean and dry. Pressure points can be covered with hydrocolloid dressings. Fragile skin at risk for breakdown can be covered with clear occlusive dressings. Foam pads, air mattresses, gel mattresses, or air-flotation beds may be necessary to minimize pressure points on cachectic patients.

When pressure ulcers do occur, they should be appropriately staged and treated. The reader should see treatment guidelines for pressure ulcers from the Agency for Healthcare Research and Quality at its website, http://www.ahrq.gov/clinic/cpgsix.htm).

Odors from superficial infection of ulcers or exophytic malignancies are usually the result of anaerobic infections and/or poor hygiene. Topical metronidazole or silver sulfadiazine bid or tid can be effective. Dakin's solution, a dilute bleach solution—0.25 percent sodium hypochlorite—can also be effective in limiting odors from anaerobic infections. Other measures that may be effective in controlling odors include placing a pan of cat litter or activated charcoal under the bed, improving room ventilation, placing an open cup of vinegar in the room, or burning a candle in the room. Adding additional fragrances in an attempt to mask odors should be avoided as it often simply leads to a repugnant concoction of odors.

Insomnia

Insomnia is a bothersome symptom for both dying patients and their families or caregivers. Foremost among general management principles is good sleep hygiene. This includes avoiding staying in bed when awake if possible, avoiding caffeine late in the day and alcohol at bedtime, and avoiding overstimulation in the hours before bedtime. Pain management is essential; long-acting medications are preferred, to control pain through the night. Some patients may benefit from using relaxation and imagery.

Pharmacologic agents that are beneficial include antihistamines, benzodiazepines, neuroleptics, and sedating antidepressants. Some examples and suggested doses are listed in table 3.5. Chlorpromazine is a more sedating agent than risperidone or haloperidol.

Table 3.5. Medications for Insomnia

MEDICATION	DOSE	ROUTE OF ADMINISTRATION / FREQUENCY
diphenhydramine	25-50 mg	PO q hs
lorazepam	0.5-2.0 mg	PO q hs
zolpidem	5-10 mg	PO q hs
risperidone or haloperidol	1 mg	PO q hs
chlorpromazine	10-100 mg	PO q hs
trazodone	25-200 mg	PO q hs
temazepam	15-45 mg	PO q hs

Source: Adapted from Common physical symptoms. In: Emanuel LL, von Gunten CF, Hauser JM, eds. The Education in Palliative and End-of-Life Care (EPEC) Curriculum. Chicago: The EPEC Project; 1999, 2003.

Conclusion

Along with a holistic approach to the general care of the dying person focusing on the individual's values and goals, careful attention to symptom control and alleviating suffering is rewarding, albeit challenging at times. It is important to educate both patients and their families/caregivers about potential symptoms and their amenability to treatment as the end of life approaches. Minimizing or eliminating symptoms maximizes comfort and can help patients feel better in spite of progressive disease and gradual decline as they near death.

Notes

1. Hockley JM, Dunlop R, Davies RJ. Survey of distressing symptoms in dying patients and their families in hospital and the response to a symptom control team. *BMJ (Clin Res Ed)*. 1988;296(6638):1715–1717.

2. LeGrand SB, Khawam EA, Walsh D, Rivera NI. Opioids, respiratory function, and dyspnea. *Am J Hosp Palliat Care*. 2003;20(1):57–61.

3. De Peuter S, Van Diest I, Lemaigre V, Verleden G, Demedts M, Van den Bergh O. Dyspnea: The role of psychological processes. *Clin Psych Rev*. 2004;24(5):557–581.

4. Foral PA, Malesker MA, Huerta G, Hilleman DE. Nebulized opioids use in COPD. *Chest*. 2004;125(2):691–694.

5. Common physical symptoms. In: Emanuel LL, von Gunten CF, Hauser JM, eds. The Education in Palliative and End-of-Life Care (EPEC) Curriculum. Chicago: The EPEC Project; 1999, 2003.

6. Ibid.

7. Ibid.

8. Bruera E, Neumann CM. Management of specific symptom complexes in patients receiving palliative care. *Canadian Med Assoc J*. 1998;158(13):1717–1726.

9. Ibid.

Part 2
The Needs of Special Populations

4
Questions and Answers about Hospice: A Guide for Physicians
Steven Zweig and Paul Tatum

The idea that dying is a natural part of life conflicts with the medicalization of death to which we have become accustomed.[1] However, all would agree that it would be inappropriate to treat only the disease of the dying patient. We would be remiss to ignore the familial, social, cultural, and spiritual dimensions of dying.

Disease-oriented care focuses solely on prolonging life, whereas comfort and quality of life are at the heart of palliative care. Palliative care is the foundation for hospice services, although palliative care may be administered in any health-care setting, not just within hospice. The word *hospice* derives from the Latin concept of *hospitium*, or hospitality. It was popularized by nurse and physician Dame Cicely Saunders, who founded one of the first hospices, St. Christopher's in London. Medicare, Medicaid (in most states), and most private insurance programs cover hospice services. Since the Medicare hospice benefit was introduced in 1983, millions of terminally ill Americans and their families have relied on this program of interdisciplinary comprehensive palliative care at home.

Most dying patients and their families want what hospice has to offer. A 1996 Gallup Poll showed that, should they become terminally ill, 88 percent of adults would prefer to be cared for in their own homes or that of a family member rather than in a hospital.[2] A similar study of cancer patients in 2003 showed that nearly 90 percent would prefer to die at home.[3] Unfortunately, 75 percent of Americans do not know that hospice care can be provided in the home, and 90 percent are unaware that hospice care can be fully covered by Medicare.[4] Nearly 2.4 million Americans died in 2007; about 930,000 of them (39 percent) received hospice care.[5] About 50 percent of Americans who die each year die in hospitals, 25 percent in nursing homes, and 25 percent in their own homes or elsewhere. Of all the deaths of patients in hospice programs in 2007, 70 percent took place in the patients' places of residence, which could be private residences, nursing facilities, or residential facilities. Only 9 percent of hospice patients died in acute-care hospitals.[6]

Hospice care is guided by an individualized plan developed by an interdisciplinary team, including a physician medical director, nurse, chaplain, social worker, and the patient's attending physician, using a comprehensive case-management approach. The goal is the creation of a care plan consistent with the preferences of the patient and designed to manage pain and other symptoms, as well as providing social support to the patient and the family. This chapter will answer some frequently asked questions about hospice and what it can provide.

What services are provided under the hospice benefit?

Under the direction of the attending physician, hospice provides the following:

- Registered nurses, often with special training in end-of-life care, furnish direct patient care and case management. The hospice nurse visits the patient as needed and is on call twenty-four hours a day for support of the patient and family.
- A medical social worker assesses needs and delivers social and instrumental support to the patient and family.

- A chaplain provides pastoral care assessment and spiritual support as desired by the patient and family members.
- The medical director supplies oversight and consultation to the multidisciplinary team and to the attending physician if desired.
- Trained hospice volunteers offer listening and companionship to the patient and family.
- Home health-care and homemaker services are also available, as are dietary counseling and ultimately bereavement support.
- Physical-, occupational-, and speech-therapy services are also available when included in the patient's written plan of care.

One thing hospice does not supply is a twenty-four-hour, in-home caregiver. In fact, to be eligible for hospice, a dependent patient must have a designated caregiver, who could be a family member or not.

Hospice services are primarily designed for caring for the dying at the patient's site of residence, whether in the home, an assisted-living center, or a nursing home. There are, in fact, four levels of hospice care under the hospice benefit:

- **Routine home care:** Standard hospice services as above are provided at the patient's residence.
- **Respite care:** Five days of respite within a hospice unit or skilled-nursing facility are available to provide relief to caregivers. This can be repeated as needed.
- **General inpatient care:** For severe, unrelenting symptoms that require more intensive management, the hospice patient may be admitted to a dedicated hospice inpatient unit or, when such a facility is not available, placed in a contracted hospital bed or skilled-nursing unit that can provide twenty-four-hour RN-level care.
- **Continuous care:** Occasionally, when the patient is near the end of life and extra services are needed to keep him

or her at home, the hospice can mobilize around-the-clock care, including RN services for symptom management.

Does hospice provide drugs and medical equipment?

Yes, as needed for palliation and management of the terminal condition. The patient is responsible for a 5 percent drug copayment, not to exceed five dollars per drug each month. Durable medical equipment such as commode chairs, walkers, and hospital beds are also supplied without charge as needed.

Who is eligible for hospice?

The short answer is: hospice is for anyone who is dying. However, it is more complicated than that. Most private insurance programs and Medicaid have a hospice benefit plan with admission guidelines resembling those of Medicare. For eligibility under the Medicare hospice benefit, a patient must

- Be eligible for Medicare Part A (Hospital Insurance).
- Have an attending physician and the hospice medical director certify that the patient has a life-limiting illness and that if the disease runs its normal course, death may be expected in six months or less.
- Sign a statement choosing hospice care instead of routine Medicare-covered benefits for the illness.
- Receive care from a Medicare-approved hospice program.

While hospice care in the United States originally went mostly to patients with cancer, in 2007 cancer patients made up only 41 percent of all hospice admissions. Patients can use hospice services with any terminal diagnosis, including chronic obstructive pulmonary disease, HIV/AIDS, congestive heart failure, renal failure, stroke, or advanced dementia. More than 80 percent of hospice patients in 2007 were Medicare recipients, but patients can enter hospice at any age. The American Academy of Hospice and Palliative Medicine has developed general and disease-specific guidelines for hospice enrollment.[7]

Do I relinquish care of my patient when he or she enters hospice?

No. During the provision of all hospice services, the attending physician remains in charge. He or she works cooperatively with the hospice interdisciplinary team, but remains responsible for the services provided and bills accordingly (see *How do I bill . . . ?* below). It is important to both physician and patient to continue their relationship during this difficult time; not only does it provide comfort to the patient, but the physician can expand his or her personal and professional expertise by guiding the hospice team. The attending physician provides orders for the personalized care plan, which should be based on goals of palliation rather than disease-oriented treatment. The hospice medical director may make suggestions to the attending physician based on the biweekly interdisciplinary team meeting, but the care of the patient remains at the discretion of the attending physician.

Some primary physicians who refer patients to hospice may prefer not to oversee their care. Sometimes the subspecialist who has been caring for the patient—an oncologist, cardiologist, or neurologist, for example—may continue as the patient's physician under hospice. If the primary physician wants to stop being involved after hospice certification, the patient can be referred to a colleague or cared for by the hospice medical director, who then acts as the attending physician.

How will hospice help me care for my patient?

We all recognize that as terminally ill patients approach death, they require more frequent and diverse help than is generally provided in office or hospital practices. The hospice team is structured to furnish these complex and time-consuming services and is designed to bring care to the patient who may no longer be able to travel for care. For the hospice patient with a problem, the first contact is the hospice nurse, who is available in person or on call at all times. The social worker and chaplain assess patients and caregivers on admission to hospice and as needed after that. The multidisciplinary team, including the medical director, regularly reviews the patient's care plan. This review, including recommendations for physician orders, is forwarded to the attending physician. As the end nears, hospice services are intensified. The hospice nurse goes to the home at the time of death (if not already present) and facilitates the transfer of the body to mortuary services. Immediately, and during the year after death, hospice provides bereavement services to surviving family or friends.

Do patients on hospice die sooner?

One barrier to timely referral is the misunderstanding that hospice is appropriate only for the last few days of life. However, the interdisciplinary-team process not only may impact quality of life and symptom management, but may actually prolong survival. In a study of 4,493 terminally ill patients, mean survival was twenty-nine days longer for those on hospice than for those who did not enroll. Longer survival was found within four of six of the studied disease types: heart failure, lung cancer, pancreatic cancer, and colon cancer.[8]

How can I be sure I am sending my patient to a good hospice?

To receive Medicare funding, each hospice must go through a certification process and an annual survey. In addition, the National Hospice and Palliative Care Organization has developed Standards of Practice for Hospice Programs that measure ten domains of quality care. Hospices that participate in the NHPCO are members of the Quality Partnership Program. In addition, personal and professional references are valuable. Clinical Practice Guidelines for Quality Palliative Care were developed by the National Consensus Project for Quality Palliative Care, a consortium of five leading U.S. palliative-care organizations. The guidelines, released in April 2004, are designed to help hospitals, nursing homes, hospices, and health systems that are establishing palliative-care programs. These guidelines are based on scientific evidence, clinical experience, and expert opinion.[9] The Center for Medicare and Medicaid Services in requiring hospices to focus on quality improvement. The new Conditions of Participation for hospices from December of 2008 make continuing quality improvement a requirement for every hospice. Every hospice executive director must be able to describe outcome data for pain and symptom management as well as pressure-ulcer incidence and fall rates over time. Web-based standardized comparisons, like those that exist for nursing homes, are not yet available.

How is hospice different from good home health care?

Hospice and Medicare-sponsored home care share some of the same goals: maintaining function and helping patients stay at home. Sometimes home health agencies also provide hospice services. Clients of Medicare-sponsored home care are expected to improve, and service ends if and when the patient stabilizes and no longer needs skilled-nursing or rehabilitative services. Most home health agencies do not have active medical director support, most do not provide pastoral care, and none supply bereavement support on a formal basis. Medicare-sponsored home health care requires that the patient be homebound, while hospice has no such requirement.

If my patient is in hospice, does that mean I can't treat pneumonia?

The short answer is no. In making a decision about treating an acute illness, one should always compare that decision with the patient's goals for care. Once a patient is in hospice, the goals of care shift from disease-oriented treatment to managing symptoms, increasing comfort, and improving quality of life. If treating pneumonia accomplishes those goals, then such treatment would be appropriate. However, near death, pneumonia may be the terminal event, and the more appropriate treatment might include antipyretics, morphine, and oxygen for managing the symptoms of fever, pain, and dyspnea, rather than antibiotics.

What if my patient doesn't die within the six-month period after admission to hospice?

Many physicians are reluctant to refer patients to hospice, concerned that they might be underestimating their length of life. In 2007, the average length of service was 67.4 days, and the median was 20 days.[10] Three months after enrollment, again three months later, then at two-month intervals thereafter, the hospice must certify that the patient continues to meet hospice criteria and can benefit from hospice services. It is unusual but not impossible for patients to live for years after enrolling in hospice as long as they continue to have an expected prognosis of six months or less.

Physicians dislike predicting when a patient's life will end, and research has shown that they are not very good at it.[11] Unfortunately, in 2007, 31 percent of patients served by hospice died in seven days or less, sometimes only hours after referral, thus preventing them from receiving the benefits that the hospice team could offer.

Physicians whose patients live longer than six months in hospice do not risk charges of Medicare fraud or abuse.

Hospice medical directors are responsible for reevaluation of prognosis in patients with extended length of stay, and they may make visits to reassess prognosis.

What if my patient wants to opt out of hospice, recovers, and doesn't need hospice?

At any time, the patient can opt out of the hospice program and go back to receiving usual Medicare benefits. Should the need arise, the patient could reenter hospice when appropriate.

What happens if my patient or the family needs a break, or if symptoms cannot be controlled at home?

For overwhelmed caregivers, the hospice can provide several days of respite services, usually by placing the patient in an area nursing home with which the hospice contracts. If symptoms cannot be managed at home, the patient can be admitted to a hospital for intensive symptom management. This hospital is paid a negotiated rate by the hospice, and no break in service is required. Since the hospice team is skilled in home-based symptom management and can intensify services when necessary, it is unusual for a patient to require hospitalization.

If the patient is already in the hospital, how can hospice get involved?

It is often during hospitalization that it becomes obvious that the patient's goals of care have shifted from disease-oriented treatment to palliative care, with the primary focus on quality of life and comfort. If the patient is not likely to die in the hospital, then hospice can provide a helpful transition of care to home or another setting, with no break in care plan or service. Attending physicians and hospitals should be encouraged to work with local hospices to foster such smooth transitions.

Can hospice provide care for nursing-home residents?

Because both Medicare-sponsored skilled-nursing care and hospice are benefits paid for by Medicare Part A, no patient can receive both services simultaneously for the same diagnosis, but any non-Medicare nursing-home patient, as long as he or she meets hospice criteria, can receive hospice benefits. Payment of room and board remains the responsibility of the patient, the family, or Medicaid for eligible residents. Specially trained hospice staff and volunteers can provide many services beyond those usually offered in nursing homes. The delivery of end-of-life care occurs within the guidelines of both the nursing home and the hospice. The coordinated plan of care must designate which care and services will be provided by the nursing home and which by the hospice, in order to best respond to the needs of the patient.[12] While 28 percent of Missouri deaths occur in nursing homes,[13] only a small percentage of elderly nursing-home residents are enrolled in hospice.[14]

How do I bill for caring for patients in hospice?

Attending physicians for hospice patients bill Medicare B through their usual carrier or bill commercial insurers, by simply adding the modifier—GV to the appropriate CPT code. Physicians who are caring for problems unrelated to the hospice diagnosis use the—GW modifier when they bill. Consulting physicians who are addressing needs related to the hospice diagnosis are effectively contracting with the hospice and bill the hospice agency itself.[15]

How can I learn more about end-of-life care?

Most physicians receive little or no training in end-of-life care in medical school, but some helpful resources exist. The online End of Life/Palliative Education Resource Center hosted by the Medical College of Wisconsin offers over 200 brief summaries of common end-of-life clinical issues, called Fast Facts, which can be read quickly and provide references for further reading (http://www.eperc. mcw.edu/ff_index.htm). Physicians, nurses, and others can participate in the Education in Palliative and End-of-Life Care (EPEC) training programs or local versions of that curriculum delivered by physicians who have undergone EPEC training. (Go to www.epec.net to purchase a Participant's Handbook.) The EPEC Project's seventeen units address a variety of communication and symptom-management challenges in end-of-life care. A pocket-size handbook available for less than twenty dollars provides useful algorithms for symptom management applicable to all settings of care.[16]

Increasingly, medical journals are publishing in-depth articles on end-of-life care, such as "Perspectives on Care at the Close of Life," published in the *Journal of the American Medical Association* (and available within the topic collection at http://jama.ama-assn.org/cgi/collection/endoflife_care_palliative_medicine). The American Academy of Hospice and Palliative Medicine offers many educational resources as well, including *Primer of Palliative Care*, 4th ed., and the nine-volume physician self-education program, the UNIPAC series.

How can I find a hospice in my community?

Hospices that serve your area can be found at the website of each state's hospice association or by searching the National Hospice and Palliative Care Organization's database (http://iweb.nhpco.org/iweb/Membership/MemberDirectorySearch.aspx?pageid=3257&showTitle=1). Representatives of most hospices will be happy to come to your patient's home to answer questions and provide information.

Notes

1. McCue JD. The naturalness of dying. *JAMA*. 1995;273:1039–1043.

2. Gallup Poll. *Knowledge and Attitudes Related to Hospice Care*. Conducted for the National Hospice Association. Princeton, NJ: Gallup; 1996.

3. Tang ST. When death is imminent: Where terminally ill patients with cancer prefer to die and why. *Cancer Nurs*. 2003;26:245–51. 2003.

4. National Hospice and Palliative Care Organization. *Facts and Figures on Hospice Care in America*. Alexandria, VA: NHPCO; 2000.

5. National Hospice and Palliative Care Organization. *Facts and Figures: Hospice Care in America*. Alexandria, VA: NHPCO; 2008.

6. Ibid.

7. Standards and Accreditation Committee, Medical Guidelines Task Force. *Medical Guidelines for Determining Prognosis in Selected Non-cancer Diseases*. 2nd ed. Arlington, VA: National Hospice Organization; 1996.

8. Connor SR, Pyenson B, Fitch K, Spence C, Iwasaki K. Comparing hospice and nonhospice patient survival among patients who die within a three year window. *J Pain Symptom Manage*. 2007;33(3):238–46.

9. National Consensus Project for Quality Palliative Care. *Clinical practice guidelines for quality palliative care*. 2004. http://www.national-consensusproject.org.

10. National Hospice and Palliative Care Organization. *Facts and Figures: Hospice Care in America*. Alexandria, VA: NHPCO; 2008.

11. Christakis NA, Iwashyna TJ. Attitude and self-reported practice prognostication in a national sample of internists. *Arch Intern Med*. 1998;158:2389–2395; Christakis NA, Lamont EB. Extent and determinants of error in doctors' prognoses in terminally ill patients: Prospective cohort study. *BMJ*. 2000;320(7233):469–473.

12. Keay TJ, Schonwetter RS. Hospice care in the nursing home. *Am Fam Phys*. 1998;57:491–494.

13. Teno J. Brown site of death atlas of the U.S. 2000. http://www.chcr.brown.edu/dying.

14. Oliver DP, Porock D, Zweig S, Rantz M, Petroski G. Hospice and nonhospice nursing home residents. *J Palliat Med*. 2003;6(1):69–75.

15. Von Gunten CF, Ferris FD, Kirschner C, Emanuel L. Coding and reimbursement mechanisms for physician services in hospice and palliative care. *J Palliat Med.* 2000; 3:157–164.

16. Wrede-Seaman L. *Symptom Management Algorithms: A Handbook for Palliative Care.* Yakima, WA: Intellicard; 1999.

5
The Burden of Caregiving at the End of Life
David A. Fleming

Patients with terminal illnesses typically require the assistance of family members, significant others, and friends to avoid hospitalization and be allowed to die at home. Nonprofessional caregivers are of central importance in end-of-life care because of the ongoing, day-to-day, often minute-to-minute care and support that is needed. They provide essential care and function as liaisons to physicians and other health professionals when patients need assistance with decision making and health-care planning.

These services are not risk free for the caregiver. Assuming the responsibility of caring for loved ones at the end of life is frequently very distressing. Caregivers are at greater risk for depression, deteriorating physical health, financial difficulties, and premature death.[1] Caregivers are also less likely to engage in preventive health behaviors or otherwise attend to their own health needs, placing them at risk for deterioration of existing chronic health problems.[2]

Caregivers add a critical dimension to care that deserves recognition and validation. Physicians and others caring for patients with terminal illness often overlook the needs of caregivers and may fail to recognize their importance. The patient, family, and caregiver coalesce into a single "unit of care" that serves to reformulate and enhance the relationship grounded in trust that forms between patients and physicians. Mutual trust and understanding between patients and their physicians are critical elements for successful end-of-life care, and the caregiver becomes an equal stakeholder in this trust relationship.

In this chapter I will underscore the importance of caregiving as a valuable part of end-of-life care and emphasize the critical importance of physicians' and other team members' being sensitive and responsive to caregiver needs. I will also review recent research that has identified factors and physician behaviors most important to caregivers during the final months of patients' lives and into bereavement. Early recognition of these factors may enable interventions that will be beneficial to the caregivers as well as their patients.

The Importance of Caregiving

In the United States cancer is the most frequent terminal illness requiring caregiving.[3] In the early 1990s it was estimated that six million people in this country had a history of cancer, and three million had had the diagnosis for over five years.[4] More than half a million people die of cancer here each year. This number will rise because cancer rates increase with age and the population is aging.[5] Many cancer patients are now being cared for at home. As the population ages and health-care systems move toward earlier discharge from hospitals, the care of more cancer patients is shifting to home and other outpatient settings. Family caregivers for terminally ill patients are also necessary because of limited support and coverage by insurers for hospice and other home health-care services.

In addition to rising cancer rates, the aging of our population also is creating a greater need for home caregivers. In the United States, overall life expectancy increased from 70.8 years in 1970 to 75.8 years in 1995.[6] One implication of this phenomenon is that within fifty years, the number of cancer diagnoses is expected to double.[7] Other forms of terminal illness will also be increasingly prevalent due to an aging population. Approximately 360,000 new cases of Alzheimer's disease are being diagnosed annually, and the prevalence doubles every five years beyond the age of sixty-five.[8]

A study of Midwest caregivers revealed that most live with their patients, and most live in rural areas or smaller communities; only one-third live in urban populations of 50,000 or more.[9] Awareness of this is important for health agencies in rural areas, where resources may be strained to support the increasing needs of terminal patients, caregivers, and physicians.

The Risks and Economic Impact of Caregiving

Most caregivers are older spouses or middle-aged adult children of severely disabled patients, and the majority of caregivers are women. Spouses have an increased mortality rate during the first year following the death of their mates,[10] and this risk is further elevated when the spouse has served as the primary caregiver during the end-of-life period. The loss of a loved one, chronic emotional distress, the physical demands of caregiving, and the biological vulnerability of older adults combine to increase the risk for health problems and early death in caregivers, especially if they are elderly. Schulz and Beach found that mortality risks were 63 percent higher in elderly caregivers who were experiencing distress, compared to those who were providing care but did not feel stressed.[11] Caregivers who live with the care recipient tend to experience higher levels of strain and burden, so this puts them at increased risk.

Very few dying patients receive paid nursing care in addition to family assistance; this implies a substantial financial burden on unpaid caregivers. It is estimated by the National Center for Health Statistics that over fifty-four million Americans serve as caregivers for chronically ill or disabled family members.[12] Most caregivers are female family members. Of caregivers, 43 percent have a household income of less than $30,000, and 54 percent are between the ages of thirty-five and sixty-four years—the primary wage-earning years. Household income, often from two wage earners, is frequently jeopardized as family members sacrifice employment to stay home and care for totally dependent loved ones.

The importance of caregiver services has historically been underrecognized and undervalued economically. Nonprofessional caregiving has been estimated to be worth $196 billion a year, while the annual expenditure for commercial home health and nursing-home care totals $32 billion and $83 billion, respectively.[13] As the number of caregivers rises, the impact of caregiving will become increasingly evident, with important social and economic implications.

The Unmet Needs of Caregivers

Caregivers living with their patients have more personal needs than caregivers who do not live with their patients.[14] The majority of patients with terminal illness report a need for assistance, but relatively few receive assistance from paid caregivers.[15] Most rely on family members and friends for help with transportation, housework, nursing, and personal care. A recent study of caregivers of patients with metastatic cancer provides insight and understanding about the caregiving experience and details of the burdens and unmet needs of caregivers.[16] Findings indicate that physicians need to be attentive to patient quality-of-life issues and attempt to provide assistance. Caregivers may need help balancing caregiving with other family, financial, and work responsibilities. It is also important for physicians to communicate effectively with the patient and the caregiver and to acknowledge the importance of caregiving.

Caregivers desire that physicians pay close attention to the medical care of the patient, both on an interpersonal and at the institutional level. A caring nature and good bedside manner are consistently rated high as an important caregiver need from a physician. Feeling secure that there is effective communication about test results, diagnosis, and course of treatment, especially when more than one physician is involved, is also important to caregivers, and effective communication within health-care systems and between providers to streamline the use and transfer of medical information, billing, and scheduling is highly desired.

In fact, caregivers stress effective and compassionate communication as perhaps the most important need they have. This includes disclosure of medical information, prognosis, treatment, and discussion of care directives and the dying patient's wishes regarding future intervention. They also identified earlier involvement of palliative-care services and timelier referral to hospice care as important.

Caregivers, at the time of diagnosis and throughout the course of illness, desire information to assist them in understanding the patient's condition and making decisions about next steps in the illness. Disclosure of medical mistakes and charting errors is important to secure caregivers' trust in both the physician and the health systems in which they practice. At the organizational level, reducing errors and inconvenience through better handling of charts, x-rays, lab data, scheduling, and transportation and by eliminating the need for burdensome administrative requirements (such as having to repeatedly fill out health forms and re-register at each visit) will reduce patient and caregiver stress.

Counseling and other forms of psychological and emotional support during the illness may provide caregivers with realistic expectations of their patient's illness. These interventions also provide an opportunity to screen for depression and anxiety in caregivers. From the initial diagnosis and repeatedly during the course of illness, the physician should emphasize the importance of caregivers' seeking and accepting practical and emotional support. Involving other members of the health-care team, such as social workers, counselors, and chaplains, can be invaluable in this process.

Caregiver Trust

Trust in the physician is a primary mediator of emotional distress because it is a major predictor of patient and caregiver satisfaction.[17] Trust may be damaged when there is poor communication and inaccurate disclosure of the patient's health status. The quality of the doctor-patient relationship and the mutual trust the relationship embodies are influenced by the physician's effectiveness in communication, interpersonal relations, and the patient's and/or caregiver's perception of the physician's clinical skill, especially in the alleviation of pain and suffering.[18] Other important traits are compassion, honesty, empathy, respect, and a genuine sense of caring.[19]

Responses from caregivers about their unmet needs suggest that loss of trust can be very distressing.[20] Trust is damaged when communication fails. Honesty is of particular concern in relation to full disclosure about medical mistakes as well as about the patient's medical condition. Actual or perceived poor communication or inattentiveness to the caregiver can undermine his or her trust in the doctor's skill and reputation.

The AMA's Council on Scientific Affairs espouses a model of care that considers the caregiver and the patient as a single unit. The caregiver becomes a partner with the physician and patient.[21] During end-of-life care, the patient's caregiver naturally becomes intertwined within the physician-patient relationship, and as a valid stakeholder often becomes the ultimate surrogate decision maker for the patient. Failure to win caregiver trust or to involve caregivers in end-of-life health decisions can compromise quality of care and prevent adequate symptom relief.

Caregiver Relief

The United States is the only developed nation in the world that does not financially support caregivers. Medicare does not cover medical expenses of long-term care in nursing homes or other long-term-care facilities. In January 2000, President Bill Clinton proposed a $3,000 annual tax credit for the many families providing long-term care for a seriously ill member.[22] Unfortunately, this proposal fell victim to budget constraints and other policy issues.

In 2002, the Living Well with Fatal Chronic Illness Act was introduced in the U.S. House of Representatives (HR 5139). This bill would have allowed a Medicare buy-in option for caregivers over fifty-five years of age and a $3,000 tax credit for the primary caregiver of a low-income individual who has long-term-care needs.[23] A similar Medicare waiver provision for caregivers already exists in some states. While such a tax credit would fall short of completely covering the financial costs incurred by many caregivers, having it available would at least demonstrate support for the significant commitment and contributions made by those who help loved ones who are dying. Additionally, HR 5139 would have authorized the Department of Health and Human Services to establish research, demonstration, and education programs to improve the quality of end-of-life care across multiple federal agencies, and it would have authorized the Department of Veterans Affairs to develop and implement similar programs for thousands of disabled veterans.

It was estimated that HR 5139 would cost over $1.5 billion a year, and it did not pass in 2002; it has not been reintroduced. To date, the political environment has not been accepting of legislation with such broad implications for social relief. However, the fact that such a bill was even introduced is evidence that the needs of caregivers are being recognized to some extent and that relief measures for such vulnerable populations may be on the horizon in our society.

Conclusion

The unmet needs of caregivers of terminally ill and chronically disabled patients are a burgeoning problem.

Caregivers benefit by having their important role recognized and validated by the health-care team and by receiving direct communication from their patients' physicians. Physicians should be sensitive and knowledgeable about caregiver burden so they can be equipped to identify caregivers at risk in the months preceding death, as well as in the early weeks and months of bereavement following the death of their patients.

Specialists who treat patients with terminal illness are positioned to recognize and implement steps necessary to alleviate caregiver distress. Primary-care physicians play a particularly important role in addressing these issues, however, because caregivers may seek assistance from their personal physicians for physical and emotional health problems while they are still in the caregiving role or during bereavement.

The World Health Organization confirms that the caregiver and patient should be considered a single unit in the relationship they form with the physician.[24] This means that caregivers have an equal stake in discussions about treatment, prognosis, and heath-care planning. Physicians should therefore be simultaneously sensitive to the needs of patients and the needs of their caregivers. Open and honest communication, including thoughtful listening to caregivers' opinions, is very important. Recognition and validation of the caregiving role, compassionate bedside manner, and attention to caregiver quality-of-life issues also contribute to caregiver support and to consolidating the trust relationship that forms between the physician, the patient, and the caregiver. Giving unique attention to caregivers' psychological needs, including early referral to appropriate services, may be vital to protecting the welfare of this important member of the health-care team.

Notes

1. Schulz R, Beach S. Caregiving as a risk factor for mortality: The caregiver health effects study. *JAMA*. 1999;282:2215–2219.

2. Schultz R, Newsom J, Mittelmark M, et al. Health effects of caregiving: The caregiver health effects study. An ancillary study of the cardiovascular health effects study. *Ann of Behavioral Med.* 1997;19:110–116.

3. Emanuel E, Fairclough D, Slutsman J, et al. Assistance from family members, friends, paid care givers, and volunteers in the care of terminally ill patients. *NEJM.* 1999;341(13):956–963.

4. Hileman J, Lackey N, Hassanein R. Identifying the needs of home caregivers of patients with cancer. *Onc Nurs Forum.* 1992;19(5):771–777.

5. Ingham J. The epidemiology of cancer at the end of life. In: Berger A, Shuster J, Van Roem J, et al., eds. *Principles and Practice of Supportive Oncology.* Philadelphia: Lippincott-Raven; 1998:749–765.

6. Rosenberg H, Ventura S, Maurer J, et al. Births and deaths: United States, 1995. In: *Monthly Vital Statistics Report.* Hyattsville, MD: National Center for Health Statistics; 1996:45(Suppl 21):1–40.

7. Edwards B, Howe H, Ries L, et al. Annual report to the nation on the status of cancer, 1973–1999, featuring implications of age and aging on U.S. cancer burden. *Cancer.* 2002;94(10):2766–2792.

8. Brookmeyer R, Gray S, Kawas C. Projections of Alzheimer's disease in the United States and the public health impact of delaying disease onset. *Am J of Pub Health.* 1998;88(9):1337–1342.

9. Ibid.

10. Mor V, McHorney C, Sherwood S. Secondary morbidity among the recently bereaved. *Am J of Psych.* 1986;143:158–163.

11. Schulz, Beach. Caregiving as a Risk Factor. Vitaliano, P. Physiological and physical concomitants of caregiving: Introduction to special issue. *Ann of Behavioral Med.* 1997;19:75–77; Kiecolt-Glaser J, Glaser R, Gravenstein S, et al. Chronic stress alters the immune response to influenza virus vaccine in older adults. *Proc of the Natl Acad of Sci U.S.A.* 1996;93:3043–3047.

12. U.S. Department of Health and Human Services. National survey of families and households. Informal caregiving: Compassion in action. June 1998.

13. Arno C, Levine C, Memmott M. The economic value of informal caregiving. *Health Affairs.* 1999;18:182–188.

14. Hileman J, Lackey N, Hassanein R. Identifying the needs of home caregivers of patients with cancer. *Onc Nurs Forum.* 1992;19(5):771–777.

15. Emanuel E, Fairclough D, Slutsman J, et al. Assistance from family members, friends, paid care givers, and volunteers in the care of terminally ill patients. *NEJM*. 1999;341(13):956–963.

16. Mangan P, Taylor K, Yabroff R, Fleming D, Ingham J. Caregiving at the end of life: Unmet needs and potential solutions. *Ann of Behavioral Med*. 2002;24(Spring):Supplement:S169.

17. Thom D. Further validation and reliability testing of the trust in physician scale. *Med Care*. 1999;37(5):510–517.

18. Safran D, Montgomery J, Chang H, et al. Switching doctors: Predictors of voluntary disenrollment from a primary physician's practice. *J Fam Practice*. 2001;50(2):130–136; Hanson L, Danis M. What is wrong with end of life care? Opinion of bereaved family members. *J Am Geriatr Soc*. 1997;45:1339–1344.

19. Thom D. Patient-physician trust: An exploratory study. *J Fam Practice*. 1997;44(2):169–176.

20. Kiecolt-Glaser J, Glaser R, Gravenstein S, et al. Chronic stress alters the immune response to influenza virus vaccine in older adults. *Proc of the Natl Acad of Sci U.S.A.* 1996;93:3043–3047.

21. American Medical Association, Council on Scientific Affairs. Physicians and family caregivers: A model of partnership. *JAMA*. 1993;269(10):1282–1284.

22. Clinton to propose aid for caregivers. *Washington Post*. January 19, 2000:A2.

23. Oberstar introduces bill on fatal chronic illness care. July 16, 2002. http://www.house.gov/oberstar/caregiver.htm.

24. World Health Organization. Cancer pain relief and palliative care. *Technical Report Series 804*. Geneva, Switzerland: World Health Organization; 1990:1–75.

6

Helping Older Patients and Their Families Make Decisions about End-of-Life Care

Steven Zweig and David R. Mehr

Most people who live to old age die from chronic disease. Three chronic diseases are the leading causes of death in people over age sixty-five: cancer, heart disease, and cerebrovascular disease. Following these are chronic and acute lower-respiratory diseases, diabetes, and Alzheimer's-type dementia. In Missouri, as in other states, 76 percent of those who die are sixty-five or older. Most people die in hospitals (55 percent), more than a quarter in nursing homes, and a smaller number at home or elsewhere.[1] So most people die after the age of sixty-five and of a chronic disease in a hospital or nursing home. Therefore, most people, with help from their families, end up facing decisions in their old age about the care they receive when they are dying.

Modern medicine is based on principles of diagnosis and treatment. In fact, all of medical education and training for resident physicians centers on these two areas, regardless of specialty. However, since most older people die of acute manifestations of chronic disease, for their physicians, elements of prognosis become more important than those of diagnosis. Furthermore, physicians often behave as if our interventions are equally effective for a specific diagnosis regardless of prognosis. Outcomes from specific interventions will vary greatly depending on the prior status of the patient; for example, cancer chemotherapy is variably beneficial depending on the functional status of the patient. In fact, if we are to incorporate an outcomes-oriented approach to clinical decision making into a broader, patient-oriented approach, we must discuss prognosis, patient preferences, and prioritization of goals before deciding on a management plan (treatment).

Since most older patients die with chronic illness, advance care planning is relevant and its goals important. The first goal is to ensure that when the patient has become incapable of decision making, the clinical care is in keeping with his or her preferences. Next is to improve health-care decisions by facilitating a shared process, allowing the proxy to represent the patient's interests, and to respond flexibly according to unforeseen clinical circumstances. Finally, advance care planning aspires to improve patient outcomes by decreasing the frequency of over- or undertreatment and reducing patient concerns about the burden on family members.[2]

Patient-centered medical decision making near the end of life includes four steps: identifying patient preferences, understanding and communicating the medical prognosis, defining goals of care, and implementing a management plan consistent with those goals.

Identifying Patient Preferences

While some people speak with their physicians or family members about what their wishes would be if they were to become seriously ill or were facing death, most do not plan for it. A relatively small percentage of people prepare a written advance directive, but even in the case of a patient who has created such a document, the accepted standard for making proxy medical decisions is to consider the question, what would she want if she were able to decide?

While the patient's wishes may not be definitely known, considering them not only shows respect for the patient, but frequently aids difficult discussions with proxies or families. A family member may be personally troubled by having to make a decision that might shorten a loved one's life, such as withholding a gastrostomy and feeding tube, but may feel more comfortable with that decision if considering it in the light of whether the patient would want to be kept alive when severely incapacitated and unable to eat.

Most states have laws that support advance care planning. For example, Missouri law validates the use of both written living wills and the naming of health-care proxies. The state's first living-will legislation was passed in 1986 and defines a living will as a person's written instructions for medical treatment, to be used if that person loses the ability to decide on such matters. The durable power of attorney for health care is a health-care proxy, someone named in writing, to make decisions when a person no longer can. A 1991 Missouri statute also permits the withholding of artificially delivered nutrition and hydration if that authority has been given in advance to the durable power of attorney for health care.

Living wills have several advantages. They extend patient self-determination and afford legal security for physicians. They may relieve patient anxiety about potential unwanted treatments. Hopefully, they promote physician-patient-family communication, reduce strife among family members, and increase physician confidence in decisions regarding withholding or withdrawing of care.

However, there are also disadvantages to living wills. Neither physicians nor patients are likely to bring up the topic for discussion. They may not be available when needed, or their whereabouts may be unknown. Furthermore, it is often difficult to know when they should be applied, which can result in inappropriate addition or withdrawal of care. Finally, a patient's wishes may change by the time the directive is brought into force.

The durable power of attorney for health care granted to a proxy may afford advantages over the living will alone. It can serve as an extension of the patient's autonomy without the need to account for all possible scenarios of dying. It formalizes our common-sense approach to patient care by enabling medical personnel to talk with an incapacitated patient's loved one or family member, one whom the patient has chosen to best represent him or her. The health-care proxy also reduces the number of people to whom the physician must respond.

But health-care proxies also have limitations. The patient may not have fully discussed his or her wishes with the proxy. This person could have an ulterior motive, or, more commonly, may not be able to accurately anticipate or represent the patient's wishes. Finally, the proxy may not be emotionally or intellectually up to the task of making difficult medical decisions about a loved one, or may demand medical treatment when there is no hope of benefit to the patient.

What are the best times to initiate these end-of-life discussions with our patients? Timothy Quill has divided these into urgent and routine indications. Urgent indications include imminent death, talk by the patient about wanting to die, inquiries about hospice or palliative care, recent hospitalization for severe progressive illness, intense suffering, and poor prognosis. Routine indications include discussing prognosis, discussing treatment with a low probability of success, talking about hopes and fears, and circumstances in which the physician would not be surprised if the patient died in six to twelve months.[3] This last indication may be particularly helpful in dealing with the uncertain prognosis in many chronic conditions, such as congestive heart failure.[4] Others have found the routine exam to be an opportune time to begin gathering information about the patient's end-of-life goals and values.

Understanding and Communicating the Medical Prognosis

To adequately inform patients about their medical condition near the end of life, physicians must be able to develop fairly accurate prognoses. Unfortunately, many studies show that we physicians are not very good at this aspect of medical practice. A recent study of hospice patients and the physicians who referred them found that the physicians predicted the patients would live, on average, more than five times longer than they actually did. The better the doctors knew the patients, the more likely they were to err in prognosis and overestimate life span.[5] The SUPPORT trial showed that just three days before death from congestive heart failure, 80 percent of patients were given a prognosis of six or more months.[6] Two days before death, 50 percent of patients with chronic obstructive lung disease were predicted to have a six-month survival.[7]

In most circumstances, neither patient nor physician wants to label the gravely ill as dying. "For most patients, two fundamental facts ensure that the transition to death will remain difficult," notes Thomas Finucane. "First is the widespread and deeply held desire to not be dead. . . . Second is medicine's limited ability to predict the future, and to give patients a precise, reliable prognosis about when death will come."[8]

However, it remains our responsibility to do our best in telling people what we know, what we have to offer in the treatment of their diseases, and what we will do to help them if those disease-oriented treatments are unsuccessful or not indicated. Cohort studies and clinical trials involving older patients with chronic illness will increasingly form our prognostic judgments. For example, one study during the last decade showed that patients with advanced dementia who are hospitalized for a hip fracture or pneumonia have a six-month mortality of over 50 percent.[9]

Defining Goals of Care

In describing our general discomfort in talking about dying, Quill describes end-of-life discussions with seriously ill patients as addressing the "elephant in the room."[10] He suggests that physicians ask patients the following questions about their goals of care in order to understand those goals and help patients achieve them:

- "Given the severity of your illness, what is most important for you to achieve?"
- "How do you think about balancing quality of life with length of life in terms of your treatment?"
- "What are your most important hopes?"
- "What are your biggest fears?"

He also recommends asking these questions about values:

- "What makes life worth living for you?"
- "Would there be any circumstances under which you would find life not worth living?"
- "What do you consider your quality of life to be now?"
- "Have you seen or been with someone who had a particularly good death or a difficult death?"

Muriel Gillick and colleagues at the Hebrew Home for the Aged in Boston have developed five pathways of care for nursing-home patients[11] that could be applied equally well to chronically ill patients at home. They prioritize the goals of care: life prolongation, maintenance of physical and cognitive function, and comfort. For those on the "Intensive Pathway," life prolongation is the prime goal, with maintenance of physical and cognitive function second, and comfort third. This pathway would employ all medical procedures, including CPR attempts, intubation, and ICU care. On the "Comprehensive Pathway," the prime goal is maintenance of physical and cognitive function, with life prolongation second, and comfort third. Attempted CPR and ICU care would likely be excluded on the Comprehensive Pathway, because they are unlikely to prolong life and may result in loss of function.

The "Basic Pathway" still has maintenance of function first, but comfort is second, and life prolongation third. This translates into nursing-home-based care or home care for all medical conditions and substitutes medical treatment for surgical treatment whenever possible. On the "Palliative Pathway," the prime goal is comfort, with the other two goals secondary. This translates to nursing-home or home-based care exclusively, with diagnostic tests kept to a minimum. For patients on the "Comfort Only" pathway, comfort is the only goal and all treatments should be directed at alleviating symptoms. Discussing comfort as a goal of care may help patients, families, and learners (students and residents) appreciate potential disadvantages of tests and treatments that at a different time of life might be considered more appropriate. For example, maintaining an intravenous line in a patient with underlying dementia with delirium has the disadvantage of requiring the use of physical restraints.

Implementing a Management Plan Consistent with the Goals of Care

The Education in Palliative and End-of-Life Care (EPEC) Curriculum defines an eight-step protocol to guide the discussion of treatment preferences, particularly when the withholding or withdrawal of a life-sustaining therapy[12] is under consideration:

1. Be familiar with policies and statutes.

Are there specific policies within hospitals or nursing homes that preclude certain medical decisions? Most states and facilities leave specific treatment decisions to the patient and physician, but you should make yourself aware of any exceptions before the need to know arises. Sometimes when facilities indicate an unwillingness to allow certain treatments to be withheld or withdrawn, their policies could be based on misunderstandings of applicable regulations.

2. Find an appropriate setting for discussion.

In the hospital, this might be a patient/family meeting when all relevant providers—physicians, nurses, social worker, and chaplain—could discuss shifting the goals of care from disease treatment to palliative care. A comfortable meeting room away from the bustle of patient-care activities is highly desirable for this gathering.

3. Determine what the patient wants to know and reconcile all parties' knowledge of the patient's condition.

A patient, his or her family, and members of the healthcare team all may have very different perceptions of the patient's condition and prognosis. These must be reconciled if a patient-centered plan is to be developed. Furthermore, for cultural or other reasons, specific discussions about death and dying may not be acceptable to some (see Chapter 7, "Cultural Sensitivity in End-of-Life Discussions"). It is important to know what kinds of information the various participants want to have and who will make what decisions.

4. Discuss general goals of care.

Plans for treatment should be consistent with patient preferences and goals of care. New circumstances may require a reconsideration of whether comfort care has assumed a more prominent role compared to other goals.

5. Establish the context of the discussion.

Reviewing the course of the illness and the range of treatment options, even if cure is not possible, may help frame the discussion for patients and families. Physicians in this position often ask the question, do you want us to do everything we can? Unfortunately, *everything* sometimes includes futile disease-oriented treatment and may even exclude important aspects of palliative care.

6. Discuss specific treatment preferences.

Be as specific as possible when asking what the patient and family prefer in terms of treatment. Use language that patients and their family members will understand. Pause frequently to check for comprehension, write things down, and be willing to clarify. Describe each possible treatment (whether a life-sustaining procedure or a specific palliative measure), and discuss the problem the treatment would address, what the treatment involves, what is likely to happen if the patient decides not to have the treatment, the benefits of the treatment, and the potential complications and burdens created by the treatment. The specifics may include no resuscitation attempts, refusal of surgical procedures or dialysis, and/or no future hospitalizations.

7. Respond to emotions.

Physicians should acknowledge the anxiety and grief that are usually associated with discussions of dying. During these emotionally charged discussions, the physician should pause frequently, assess the participants' feelings, and respond to those feelings. When emotions are clearly evident, the physician can address them directly (saying, for example, "You seem to be very sad"). Asking questions about perceived feelings (for example, "Are you feeling angry?") is a safe way to approach a patient or family member whose emotions are not immediately identifiable. Physicians should not hesitate to get assistance from pastoral counselors or other members of the health-care team in handling these emotional discussions.

8. Establish a plan.

Finally, seek to establish a plan that is well formulated and understood by all. This may include transfer of setting of care, specific withholding or withdrawal of care, and deciding when to meet again.

Experiences of Dying

Each experience of death is unique. However, a few well-defined chronic-illness trajectories encompass a large number of dying older patients. We have selected four to discuss further.

The patient with chronic heart or lung disease who has frequent acute-illness exacerbations. The chronic nature of these diseases affords ample opportunity to review patient preferences and goals of care. Both conditions require expert medical management and patient-caregiver collaboration to maintain maximum function. Prognosis is especially difficult, since patients will typically exhibit several (possibly many) cycles of becoming acutely ill and then at least partially recovering after intensive medical interventions. Their decline is not steady, as is often the case with a dying cancer patient. The SUPPORT study showed that death can come suddenly and unexpectedly to these patients.[13]

Continuing to discuss patient preferences is imperative. The patient who may have started on the Intensive Pathway, in which life prolongation is the prime goal, may over time decide that the primary focus should be shifted to function and comfort. Here interventions such as attempted CPR and intubation must be discussed early on—decisions about whether or not to hospitalize again become important as the goals of care shift.

Attention to managing symptoms such as dyspnea and fatigue eventually becomes more relevant than treating the underlying disease. Hospice referral may be appropriate,

not only to provide symptom management, but also to support at home or in a nursing home those who have decided
not to go back to the hospital. In considering the possibility
of hospice referral, asking whether death would be surpris-
ing within six months or a year may be useful to help deal
with our own difficulties in prognostication, as well as with
patients' reluctance to face that death may be near. Also, it
may be helpful to give patients and families the opportunity to focus on specific measures to enhance comfort.

The patient with an incurable malignancy. Like patients with congestive heart failure or chronic obstructive
pulmonary disease, those with incurable malignancies may
retain cognitive capacity until the very end. Since cancer
usually progresses slowly, this means that eliciting patient
preferences along the way and regularly reviewing goals of
care in the context of prognosis is critically important. As
with the chronic heart- or lung-disease patient, several physicians may be caring for the patient simultaneously. Older
patients and family members may find the disease-oriented
treatments confusing, so it is important that specialists col-
laborate with the primary-care physician, who can coordinate care and facilitate communication.

Plans of care should include symptom management: the
average cancer patient suffers from ten different symptoms
during the course of the illness.[14] Dying of cancer is the model upon which the current Medicare hospice benefit is based.
If referrals are made in a timely fashion, symptoms (as well
as the social and spiritual needs of patients and family members) can be addressed from a multidisciplinary perspective.

The patient with end-stage dementia. Excluding diseases that can masquerade as dementia, all true dementias
are progressive and inexorably result in cognitive decline,
functional loss, and death. Pharmaceuticals (such as the
cholinesterase inhibitors) designed to treat dementia, primarily Alzheimer's disease, may slow decline, but do not
stop it. Thus, it is crucial that patients communicate treatment preferences and name a health-care proxy early in

the course of the disease. Since the disease has expected outcomes, preferences can be elicited early on about specific interventions, such as resuscitation attempts, hospitalization, treatment of infections, and artificially delivered nutrition and hydration. However, most patients at present do not create advance directives while they are competent, nor are they represented by legally appointed guardians. In such cases, family members typically are called upon to reach decisions about care. In discussing care with family members, it is particularly important to help them keep in mind the perspective of the patient as if he or she were able to decide.

Many patients with dementia eventually are admitted to nursing homes. Such patients might appropriately enter the palliative pathway. This translates into nursing home–based care exclusively, with diagnostic tests kept to a minimum. Hospitalization might appropriately be restricted to situations in which comfort would be compromised in the nursing home (for example, in some cases of hip fracture). For these patients, CPR is extremely unlikely to be of benefit,[15] and Finucane and colleagues, as well as Gillick, have persuasively argued that tube feeding has limited value.[16]

In end-stage dementia, when the patient can no longer communicate, ambulate, or sustain adequate oral nutrition, comfort care might become the only goal. That is, pneumonia would be treated with oxygen, antipyretics, and morphine, but not antibiotics. In the population with severe dementia who are hospitalized, Sean Morrison and Albert Siu have demonstrated very high six-month mortality.[17] While some family members may feel that any care limitation is inappropriate even considering the patient's preferences, many others will welcome being approached by the physician about care limitations.

The patient with an unexpected catastrophic decline. Major traumas and unexpected catastrophic illnesses also occur in older adults. A good example is severe stroke, where there are several issues. First, the extent of potential recovery may be unclear for several days or even weeks. Therefore, long-term decisions may need to be deferred for a period of time, and some aggressive measures, such as mechanical ventilation or enteral tube feeding, may need to be instituted with the understanding that they can be discontinued later. Setting time limits for reconsidering care is particularly important in this setting. We do know that there are some indicators that help predict prognosis for these patients. For example, people over eighty years old with an ischemic stroke have a 52 percent risk of dying within one year, and those who survive tend to suffer severe disability.[18] A patient with impaired consciousness, dysphagia, and urinary incontinence has a 75 percent chance of dying within thirty days after a stroke.[19]

Second, particularly in the frail elderly, a catastrophic illness may be accompanied by multiple interacting organ failures. Consider a patient admitted from a nursing home with mild dementia who then sustains a stroke with hemiparesis, developing aspiration pneumonia, delirium, and progressive renal insufficiency. Previously recorded advance care directives may not address such a situation. While the prognosis for each of this patient's problems individually may be good, together they create a significant risk for prolonged intensive care and inevitably worsening functional status.

All such catastrophic illnesses require close communication with key family members or the health-care proxy, if one is appointed. Circumstances can change quickly, and difficult treatment decisions may have to be made, including whether to attempt CPR, intubate, give parenteral or enteral nutrition, and even begin dialysis. Being clear in stating that initiated care can later be withdrawn may be particularly helpful at such times.

Having a script like the following to initiate CPR discussions can be helpful:

"If your mother were to die suddenly, that is, she stopped breathing or her heart stopped, we could try to revive her by using cardiopulmonary resuscitation (CPR). Are you familiar with CPR? Have you given any thought as to whether she would want it? Given the severity of your mother's illness, CPR would likely be ineffective. I would recommend that we choose not to attempt it, but that we continue with all other potentially effective treatments. What do you think?"[20]

This example is particularly notable in that the physician states an opinion and asks for input from family members. Due to their relative inexperience and lack of medical knowledge, family members are almost always at a disadvantage, even after extensive discussions. We believe that in most circumstances it is cruel to simply pose choices to family members without the physician's stating his or her opinion and then asking for input. Family members should not be placed in the position of feeling that *they* have to choose between death or an unproductive life for their loved one.

Conclusion

Unquestionably, there are barriers to discussing end-of-life care with patients and their families. Uncertain prognosis and gradual decline may leave optimum decision points unclear. Physicians may be uncomfortable initiating potentially difficult and time-consuming discussions. Nonetheless, it is usually beneficial to address these issues before a crisis occurs, when treatment decisions must be made quickly.

Physicians can do a great deal to help elderly patients and their family members make decisions regarding end-of-life care. Most people who die are old, and most old people die of chronic diseases, so our traditional approach to clinical decision making—which includes only diagnosis and treatment—is insufficiently oriented toward achieving best outcomes and fulfilling patient desires. A four-step process to achieving patient-centered decision making about end-of-life issues includes eliciting patient preferences, determining and communicating prognosis, defining goals of care, and implementing a management plan consistent with those goals. Physicians and family members who achieve the goals of care they set can acknowledge that they have helped someone experience a good death—the departure of a valued person who died comfortably, his or her physical, emotional, and spiritual needs having been fulfilled.

Notes

1. Missouri Department of Health and Senior Services, Center for Health Information Management and Evaluation. *Missouri Vital Statistics 2000.* Jefferson City, MO; 2001.

2. Teno JM, Nelson HL, Lynn J. Advance care planning: Priorities for ethical and empirical research. Special supplement. *Hastings Center Report.* 1994;24:S32-S36.

3. Quill TE. Perspectives on care at the close of life. Initiating end-of-life discussions with seriously ill patients: Addressing the "elephant in the room." *JAMA.* 2000;284(19):2502–2507.

4. Dy S, Lynn J. Getting services right for those sick enough to die. *BMJ.* 2007;334:511–513.

5. Christakis NA, Lamont EB. Extent and determinants of error in doctors' prognoses in terminally ill patients: Prospective cohort study. *BMJ.* 2000;320(7233):469–473.

6. The SUPPORT Principal Investigators. A controlled trial to improve care for seriously ill hospitalized patients: The Study to Understand Prognosis and Preferences for Outcomes and Risks of Treatment (SUPPORT). *JAMA.* 1995;274(20):1591–1598.

7. Lynn J, Harrell F Jr., Cohn F, Wagner D, Connors AF Jr. Prognoses of seriously ill hospitalized patients on the days before death: Implications for patient care and public policy. *New Horizons.* 1997;5(10):56–61.

8. Finucane TE. How gravely ill becomes dying. *JAMA.* 1999;282:1670–1672.

9. Morrison RS, Siu AL. Survival in end-stage dementia following acute illness. *JAMA.* 2000;284(1):47–52.

10. Quill TE. Perspectives on care at the close of life. Initiating end-of-life discussions with seriously ill patients: Addressing the "elephant in the room." *JAMA.* 2000;284(19):2502–2507.

11. Gillick M, Berkman S, Cullen L. A patient-centered approach to advance medical planning in the nursing home. *J Am Geriatr Soc.* 1999;47(2):227–230.

12. Withholding/withdrawing therapy. In: Emanuel LL, von Gunten CF, Hauser JM, eds. The Education in Palliative and End-of-Life Care (EPEC) Curriculum. Chicago: The EPEC Project; 1999, 2003.

13. The SUPPORT Principal Investigators. A controlled trial to improve care for seriously ill hospitalized patients: The Study to Understand Prognosis and Preferences for Outcomes and Risks of Treatment (SUPPORT). *JAMA.* 1995;274(20):1591–1598.

14. Morita T, Sunoda J, Inoue S, Chihara S. Contributing factors to physical symptoms in terminally ill cancer patients. *J Pain Symptom Manage* 1999;18.338 3 18.

15. Zweig SC. Cardiopulmonary resuscitation and do-not-resuscitate orders in the nursing home. *Arch Fam Med.* 1997;6(5):424–429.

16. Finucane TE, Christmas C, Travis K. Tube feeding in patients with advanced dementia: A review of the evidence. *JAMA.* 1999;282(14):1365–1370; Gillick MR. Rethinking the role of tube feeding in patients with advanced dementia. *NEJM.* 2000;342(3):206–210.

17. Morrison RS, Siu AL. Survival in end-stage dementia following acute illness. *JAMA.* 2000;284(1):47–52.

18. Marini C, Baldassarree M, Russo T, De Santis F, et al. Burden of first-ever ischemic stroke in the oldest old: Evidence from a population-based study. *Neurology.* 2004;62(1):77–81.

19. Wang Y, Lim L, Levi C, Heller RF, Fischer J. A prognostic index for 30-day mortality after stroke. *J Clin Epidemiology.* 2001;54:766–773.

20. Paraphrased from Quill TE. Perspectives on care at the close of life. Initiating end-of-life discussions with seriously ill patients: Addressing the "elephant in the room." *JAMA.* 2000;284(19):2506.

7
Cultural Sensitivity in End-of-Life Discussions
David A. Fleming

Encounters between physicians and patients of different cultures are increasingly common in today's diverse society. The need for cultural awareness by health-care providers is therefore becoming more important. This is especially true in end-of-life discussions, where cultural beliefs and traditions may strongly influence decisions made by patients and their families. Attitudes regarding death and dying vary significantly between countries and even between groups of different cultural backgrounds within countries.[1] Questions pertaining to disclosure of information, advance directives, assisting death, and the withholding or withdrawing of treatment are some of the major ethical challenges confronted during terminal illness that are influenced by cultural background.

Health-care professionals experienced in palliative care tend to have similar attitudes about caring for dying patients regardless of their sociocultural context.[2] This suggests that certain attitudes about death and dying are shared universally by health-care professionals in spite of the wide variation of beliefs and the typically strong influence of religion and cultural background. But these attitudes may differ markedly from those held by patients and their families.

Cultural demographics are changing dramatically in this country. The trends in growth and concentration indicate a need for greater awareness and sensitivity to the cultural needs of ethnic minorities, especially in geographic areas where expansion has been greatest. Using as an example one midwestern state, the population of Missouri increased from 5,117,073 in 1990 to 5,595,211 in 2000. Overall, Missouri's population grew by 9.34 percent, but central Missouri's grew by 14.57 percent. The African American population grew by 14.1 percent in the state, and was up 33.46 percent in central Missouri. Missouri's Hispanic population nearly doubled, increasing by 168 percent in the central corridor of the state. Though Hispanics comprise only 2.1 percent of Missouri's population, many areas of the state are densely populated due to cultural cohesiveness. In Saline County, for instance, 4.4 percent of the population is Hispanic. Asians and Native Americans make up 1.4 percent and 1.1 percent of Missouri's population, respectively, but there are some areas where the Asian population is more concentrated. In Boone County, Asians comprise 3 percent of the population.² These numbers indicate that cultural diversity is not coming to Missouri —it is already there. Similar cultural demographic shifts are occurring in other states.

With these increases in minority populations, the urgency of considering the variability of beliefs and values among patients who are dying has never been more pressing. The task of this chapter is to review the cultural perspectives that influence decisions at the end of life and to encourage clinicians to be sensitive to these influences. The risk of misunderstanding can be minimized by gaining awareness that cultural influences exist, learning about these influences, responding to these differences respectfully, and taking into account the values and beliefs of each individual patient. On the other side of the coin, cultural stereotyping can be disruptive, and consideration of this potential source of conflict reemphasizes the importance of being patient centered and maintaining good communication when dealing with end-of-life issues.

The Historical Context of Death

The ideal of helping people to "die well," with the focus on relieving pain and suffering, occupied the core of medical moral discourse for over two thousand years.[4] Death in most societies was an accepted part of life and was often welcomed as a means of escape from suffering. But the expectancy that life will lead to death has been blurred by the modern advancement of medical science. The ability to postpone death through repeated medical interventions has created unreasonable expectations of longevity, regardless of the disease, severity of illness, or prognosis. An ethical paradox has resulted. The societal emphasis on cure rather than care, and the medical emphasis on continued intervention and treatment, has led to fear by many patients that they will suffer needlessly at the end of life.[5] Today, people live longer, and at least 70 percent of Americans die in hospitals or other institutions, rather than at home.[6] Many spend their last days on life support and in critical-care settings despite their own health-care directives to the contrary.[7]

Death, once an inevitable and accepted partner of life, has become the enemy and is only "reluctantly admitted into the realm of medicine" as the most imposing barrier to achieving a longer life and an improved quality of life.[8] Induced by their fear of medical entrapment, patients are now asking for more information and demanding greater control over health-care decisions while they are still able to speak for themselves.

Discussions about end-of-life care topics, such as limiting treatment and the use of health-care directives, are now expected. Patients and families across all cultures are concerned and more aware of other options for terminally ill patients, such as palliative care and hospice. Physicians should be sensitive to the influences of cultural background when these issues arise, and recognize that verbal and written health-care directives reflect core values of patients as tempered by their cultural heritage. Physicians should also be sensitive to the influence that their own cultural background has on decision making and the advice that they give to patients during terminal illness.

In some ethnic groups, discussions about limiting treatment and assisted suicide tend to be avoided for reasons that are not always clear. For instance, African American patients are more likely to desire life-sustaining treatments and less likely to complete health-care directives or pursue palliative-care options than white patients. This tendency is not necessarily related to lack of trust or fear of inadequate medical treatment.[9]

Communicating about Death and Advance Directives

The enthronement of autonomy as *the* guiding ethical principle for health care is felt by some to be the most important achievement of the North American bioethics movement that began in the early 1970s.[10] Advance directives and full disclosure about prognosis are direct descendants of the principle of autonomy insofar as these forms of communication theoretically represent discussions about personal values, wishes, and expectations regarding decisions at the end of life. The United States has vigorously embraced a focus on individual autonomy and the use of both written and verbal advance directives that provide clear and convincing evidence as to patients' wishes when they are unable to speak for themselves.[11] Legal requirements for the implementation of health-care directives were provided in 1990 with *Cruzan v. Director, Missouri Department of Health,* the first "right to die" case to reach the United States Supreme Court, in which the state was ultimately allowed to remove a feeding tube from twenty-five-year-old Nancy Cruzan, who was in a persistent vegetative state following head trauma from a car accident. In response to *Cruzan,* the United States Congress passed the Patient Self-Determination

Act in 1991 requiring all federally funded health entities to inquire about health-care directives with every patient.[12] Such aggressive application of autonomy has not been the rule worldwide, however.

Asian, European, and Middle Eastern cultures have been less focused on informing patients about prognosis and encouraging personal choice at the end of life. These societies tend to favor dignified death, which they encourage through open discussion, but they have not ratified the use of advance directives in statute or regulation.[13]

In Japan, decisions are based on a paternalistic model whereby the physician directs care and informs the family but not the patient. Not directly informing the patient is felt to be in "the best interest of the patient" because knowing the prognosis would add to the suffering of the dying person. Asian families often take this kind of protective role in decision making, though their doing so cannot always be assumed since families will differ in their approach to these difficult periods.

The European genocide of the 1930s influenced much of the debate regarding end-of-life issues in Europe and the United States because of the greater awareness of suffering and death. In Germany, living wills and decisions by proxy are now recognized, though their implementation has not been legally ratified. Advance directives tend to be accepted, but they are viewed as guidelines that endorse patient choice. The expectation is that the physician will make the ultimate decisions.

Discussing end-of-life issues and advance directives effectively with patients and families requires physician sensitivity to their beliefs regarding disclosure of information to patients about their diseases and careful assessment of patients' expectations about life-sustaining interventions and about what mechanism is going to be used to make that decision. Though rarely used outside of the United States, written advance directives appear to make a significant difference in decision making at the end of life regardless of the cultural milieu. Patients at the end of life are more likely to undergo treatment in Asia, Europe, and the Middle East than in the United States. Interestingly, physicians from all countries have been willing to forgo these treatments if specific advance directives are in place.

Physicians should also take into account their own beliefs if they are very different from those of a patient. If ideological differences exist, this disconnect may disrupt the physician-patient relationship and cause a breakdown in communication, limiting the physician's ability to disclose certain information or to assist the patient and family in end-of-life planning. Should disruption in the relationship be imminent, referral to a different provider ought to be considered.

Autonomy and Assisting Death

Euthanasia is a merciful act that directly or indirectly causes the death of a suffering person. The intention is to end suffering, and the method chosen is as painless as possible. Assisted suicide is the prescribing of medication or otherwise providing a means by which a patient can take his or her own life. Though the Hippocratic oath proscribes any form of "mercy killing," the moral arguments for direct voluntary euthanasia and physician-assisted suicide (PAS) have become increasingly vigorous worldwide, carried forward by the autonomy movement that began in the United States in the 1970s.

A popular argument defending these practices is that it is a beneficent and compassionate thing to do for suffering patients. Equally compelling is the argument that dying patients have the right to choose when and where they will die. Physicians' respect for this choice preserves dignity by enabling personal control after patients become incapacitated.

A countervailing argument is that allowing (or requiring) a physician to take life is in violation of professional standards and will undermine trust at a crucial time in the patient-physician relationship. Others fear that social acceptance of euthanasia and PAS will diminish the intrinsic value of life and ultimately lead to the slippery slope of involuntary euthanasia for incompetent persons who are believed to be suffering or otherwise existing in a life not worth living. It is feared that choosing death may become too easy when other options for treatment and care remain viable.

In the United States, public and professional sentiments lean in favor of legalizing PAS. In the 1990s, 60 percent of physicians and nearly 70 percent of the public surveyed favored legalization of PAS.[14] Though a majority of terminally ill patients surveyed support legalization, only about 11 percent reported that they would seriously consider PAS for themselves, and about half of these later changed their minds, suggesting considerable ambivalence.[15] With increasing public pressure, five U.S. states have introduced public referenda on whether to allow PAS under specific conditions. Thus far, only Oregon and Washington have been successful in passing such a statewide referendum. On November 5, 2008, the state of Washington voted to allow legal assisted suicide based on the Oregon model. Oregon's Death with Dignity Act was passed in 1994 and became the first law anywhere in the world to legalize physician-assisted suicide.[16] In the first six years following that legalization, forty-two terminally ill patients died as a result of assisted suicide in Oregon.[17] The primary reasons given for requesting assistance were not fear of pain or physical suffering, but fear of losing control of bodily functions and the sense of autonomy.

Other societies have decriminalized these activities. On November 28, 2000, the Lower House of the Dutch Parliament, by a vote of 104–40, approved a bill to legalize euthanasia and physician-assisted suicide.[18] Though technically illegal only in 2000, euthanasia and PAS had been tolerated and practiced openly in the Netherlands for over twenty years before that, to the extent that in 1987 the Royal Dutch Association of Pharmacy had issued guidelines on the use and preparation of drugs for euthanasia.[19] By 1999, more than two thousand deaths were being reported annually in the Netherlands resulting from euthanasia and PAS, though some believe that many more such deaths have occurred but have gone unreported.[20]

Other Western societies have also allowed such practices. In May 1995, the Northern Territory of Australia legalized euthanasia, but the law was overridden within a year by the national parliament.[21] Withholding or withdrawing treatment for terminally ill patients is allowed in European countries; however, active euthanasia or assisted suicide is discouraged or forbidden in most. Switzerland is unique in that assisted suicide is illegal there only when the assisting person stands to gain personally.[22]

It is estimated that voluntary euthanasia occurs in twelve out of the forty-nine countries affiliated with the International Association for Suicide Prevention (IASP), although these acts are illegal in all. Concern for these findings prompted the IASP to investigate, and it discovered that over 20 percent of patients admitted to hospice care in Ireland have a positive attitude toward euthanasia. Not surprisingly, the majority of these patients (sixteen of twenty-two examined in one study) were found to be clinically depressed or anxious, which shows the relevance of psychological factors' influence on end-of-life decisions.[23]

Asian cultures are less inclined to promote patient choice, instead honoring the established authority of the physician, which is in marked contrast to Western opinions. The Japanese view death as "incorporation with nature and return to nature," and they believe in allowing death to occur at "Nature's hand."[24] Though suicide may be accepted as a personal choice, assisting or otherwise hastening death for someone with terminal illness is not consistent with the Asian belief that death comes naturally and in its own time.

With noted exceptions, the active and intentional ending of life is legally prohibited across Asia, the Middle East, Europe, and North America. Where it is legally permitted, however, actively assisting death is common. As many as 45 percent of Dutch physicians report that, with parental consent, they sometimes allow infants to die or actively assist their death when further treatment is felt to be futile.[25] Up to 25 percent of Dutch physicians admitted to euthanizing incompetent adult patients without their consent when treatment was clearly no longer indicated or effective.[26]

The debate about assisting death for terminally ill patients may be irreconcilable because the public demand for euthanasia services is in conflict with professional standards, even though most physicians favor legalizing PAS; and it is confronted by political resistance to legalization in most countries. But people, though culturally diverse, tend to share a common wish to avoid suffering and loss of control that is often greater than their fear of death. Awareness and sensitivity to the psychological factors that tend to encourage requests for euthanasia or assisted suicide will prepare the physician to respond when these requests are made.

Limiting Treatment

Although intentional ending of life is usually not sanctioned, when considering limiting futile treatment, there is general cross-cultural consensus that overly aggressive nonindicated treatment should be discouraged.[27] Patients and families of Asian descent tend to desire more aggressive treatment if patient preferences are not clear. When death is imminent, however, Asians encourage aggressive palliative care. In Japan, patients tend to expect physicians to intervene paternalistically to prolong life beyond what physicians in North America and Europe might do, but

Japanese physicians will also act aggressively to optimize comfort measures when it is clear that death is imminent.[28] In general, there tends to be cross-cultural agreement on decisions not to force oral or intravenous fluid on dying patients, to restrict unnecessary diagnostic procedures, to emphasize hospice care, and to use advance directives.[29] However, the treatment of incompetent elderly patients varies widely and warrants comment. One study examined medical treatment of incompetent elderly patients with life-threatening, but not necessarily terminal, illness in seven countries and found considerable variability of attitudes and behavior. Up to 40 percent of physicians chose a level of care different from what had been requested by the patient, and 10 percent would have tried CPR despite a "do not resuscitate" request. South American and United States physicians were found to be most aggressive with treatment decisions, while Australian physicians tended to be more conservative, respecting patient requests to limit treatment.[30] These findings support other studies that show conflicting attitudes in the care of critically ill elderly patients with dementia.

Inconsistent attitudes about end-of-life care may exist between ethnic groups within American society as well. African American patients tend to place a higher value on longevity and tend to request more life-sustaining treatments than white patients. African American physician attitudes follow the same pattern, bringing into question whether socioeconomic status, lack of familiarity with treatments, or lack of trust account for the difference.[31] The reason for this difference in attitude is unclear, but the historical lack of trust in this demographic must still be considered as a factor, as well as the tendency for strong religious preferences in the African American population.

The differences in opinion about treating patients with critical or terminal illness underscore the difficulty that pluralistic societies have in defining futility of treatment and quality of life. The moral algorithm of Edmund Pellegrino is useful in defining futility when the limitation or withdrawal of treatment is being considered. (See Chapter 10, "The Path Ahead: Difficult Lessons for Physicians and Society," for further discussion of Pellegrino's futility algorithm.) When there is a disproportionate relationship between the burden of further treatment and the relative sum of therapeutic effectiveness and the presumed benefits to be derived, life support may and perhaps should be withdrawn.[32] Though it is up to the clinician to determine clinical effectiveness of the treatments being considered, only the patient can ultimately determine the perceived benefits and burdens of such treatment relevant to their his or her life plan, values, and beliefs. Decisions about futility and limiting treatment are unique to each clinical encounter and must be individualized, taking into account the moral beliefs and cultural background of each patient.

Evaluating Cultural Influence

It is very important for health-care providers to avoid cultural stereotyping when assessing the potential influence that cultural background is having on patients and their families during end-of-life discussions. Though core values and beliefs may be influenced by cultural origin, how those core beliefs are developed individually must be acknowledged in order to build trust and enable open communication. Physicians can use knowledge about particular cultural beliefs, values, and practices to respectfully recognize a person's identity and to assess the degree to which a specific patient and family might adhere to their cultural background. One tool suggested to enhance the usefulness of this dialogue is for physicians to consciously evaluate five things: patients' and families' attitudes, beliefs, context, decision making, and environment ("ABCDE").[33] The purpose of this mnemonic device is to help physicians avoid the dual pitfalls of cultural ignorance and cultural stereotyping. This assessment can also serve to identify potential areas of conflict and opportunities for negotiation should conflict occur.[34]

Conclusion

Cultural origins of belief shape individuals' perception of the meanings of illness, suffering, and death. This holds true for health-care providers as well as patients. As ethnic and cultural diversity become more prominent, there will be greater risk for cross-cultural misunderstanding and communication breakdown when engaging in end-of-life discussions. It is therefore increasingly important that health care providers be able to assess the influence that cultural beliefs have on patient attitudes, and that they communicate effectively about these issues. Assessing cultural influence will help to minimize the risk of cultural stereotyping as well as cultural ignorance, and may prevent miscommunication about unwanted and potentially harmful treatment at the end of life.

Though modern medical advancements have blurred the traditional acceptance of death as being a natural part of life, since the 1970s physicians and health-care systems in all cultures have identified the importance of respecting the wishes of the patient and tend to promote palliative care and the limitation of unnecessary treatments at the end of life. Asian, Hispanic, Middle Eastern, and African American patients often expect more aggressive treatment than white people at the end of life, but they typically share in the belief that palliative care and limiting treatment are desirable when the patient's wishes are clearly known and when death is clearly imminent.

Notes

1. Caralis P, Davis B, Wright K, et al. The influence of ethnicity and race on attitudes toward advance directives, life-prolonging treatments, and euthanasia. *J Clin Ethics*. 1993;4(2):155–165.

2. Voltz R, Akabayashi A, Reese C, et al. Attitudes of healthcare professionals toward clinical decisions in palliative care: A cross-cultural comparison. *J Clin Ethics.* 1999;10(4):309–315.

3. U.S. Census Bureau, Census 2000.

4. Etziony M. *The Physician's Creed: An Anthology of Medical Prayers, Oaths, and Codes of Ethics Written and Recited by Medical Practitioners through the Ages.* Springfield, IL: Charles C. Thomas; 1973.

5. The SUPPORT Principal Investigators. A controlled trial to improve care for seriously ill hospitalized patients: The Study to Understand Prognosis and Preferences for Outcomes and Risks of Treatments (SUPPORT). *JAMA.* 1995;274(20):1591–1598.

6. Lyons J. Boomers begin looking beyond the good life to the "good death." *Wall Street Journal.* February 25, 2000.

7. The SUPPORT Principal Investigators. A controlled trial to improve care for seriously ill hospitalized patients: The Study to Understand Prognosis and Preferences for Outcomes and Risks of Treatments (SUPPORT). *JAMA.* 1995;274(20):1591–1598.

8. Callahan D. Pursuing a peaceful death. *Hastings Center Report.* 1993;(July-August):33–38.

9. Mckinley E, Garrett J, Evans A, and Danis M. Differences in end-of-life decision making among black and white ambulatory cancer patients. *J Gen Intern Med.* 1996;11:651–656.

10. Sanchez-Gonzalez MA. Advance directives outside the USA: Are they the best solution everywhere? *Theoretical Med.* 1997;18:283–301.

11. Lynn J, Teno J, Dresser R, et al. Dementia and advance-care planning: Perspectives from three countries on ethics and epidemiology. *J Clin Ethics.* 1999;10(4):271–285.

12. *Cruzan v. Director, Department of Health,* 110 S. Ct. 284 (1990); Omnibus Reconciliation Act of 1990 (OBRA-90), Pub. L. 101–508, sec. 4206 and 4751 (Medicare and Medicaid, respectively).

13. Sanchez-Gonzalez MA. Advance directives outside the USA: Are they the best solution everywhere? *Theoretical Med.* 1997;18:283–301.

14. Bachman J, Alcser K, Doukas D, et al. Attitudes of Michigan physicians and the public toward legalizing physician-assisted suicide and voluntary euthanasia. *NEJM.* 1996;334(5):303–309; Blendon R. Should physicians aid their patients in dying? The public perspective. *JAMA.* 1992;267(19):2658–2662.

15. Emanuel E, Fairclough D, Emanuel L. Attitudes and desires related to euthanasia and physician-assisted suicide among terminally ill patients and their caregivers. *JAMA*. 2000;284(19):2460–2468.

16. Oregon Death with Dignity Act, ballot measure no. 16 (November 8, 1994): Revised Statute 127.800–995 (1995).

17. Ganzini L, Lee M, Schmidt T, et al. Physicians' experiences with the Oregon Death with Dignity Act. *NEJM*. 2000;342(8):557–563.

18. Associated Press. Dutch Parliament legalizes euthanasia. *New York Times*. November 28, 2000.

19. Groenewoud J, van der Heide A, Onwauteaka-Philipsen B, et al. Clinical problems with the performance of euthanasia and physician assisted suicide in the Netherlands. *NEJM*. 2000;342(8):551–556.

20. Richburg K. Netherlands move to legalize anointed suicide. *Washington Post*. November 28, 2000.

21. Phillips P. Views of assisted suicide from several nations. *JAMA*. 1997;278(12):969–970.

22. Kelleher M, et al. IASP Task Force on Euthanasia and Assisted Suicide. *Crisis*. 1995;16(3):111–115, 120.

23. Kelleher M, et al. Euthanasia and the terminally ill: Can the civil killing of others be eroded? *Crisis*. 1998;9(3):116–118.

24. Ishiwata R, Sakai A. The physician-patient relationship and medical ethics in Japan. *Cambridge Quarterly of Healthcare Ethics*. 1994;3:60–66.

25. Van der Heide A, van der Maas P, van der Wal G, et al. Medical end-of-life decisions made for neonates and infants in the Netherlands. *Lancet*. 1997;350:251–255.

26. Hendin H, Rutenfrans C, Zylicz Z, et al. Physician-assisted suicide and euthanasia in the Netherlands: Lessons from the Dutch. *JAMA*. 1997;277(21):1720–1722.

27. McHaffe H, Cuttini M, Brölz-Voit G, et al. Withholding/withdrawing treatment from neonates: Legislation and official guidelines across Europe. *J Med Ethics*. 1999;25:440–446.

28. Ishiwata R, Sakai A. The physician-patient relationship and medical ethics in Japan. *Cambridge Quarterly of Healthcare Ethics*. 1994;3:60–66.

29. Voltz R, Akabayashi A, Reese C, et al. Attitudes of healthcare professionals toward clinical decisions in palliative care: A cross-cultural comparison. *J Clin Ethics*. 1999;10(4):309–315.

30. Alemayehu E, Molloy W, Guyatt G, et al. Variability in physicians' decisions on caring for chronically ill elderly patients: An international study. *Canadian Med Assoc J.* 1991;144(9):1133–1138.

31. Mebane E, Oman R, Kroonen L, Goldstein M. The influence of physician race, age, and gender on physician attitudes toward advance care directives and preferences for end of life decision making. *J Am Geriatr Soc.* 1999;47:579–591.

32. Pellegrino E. Decisions to withdraw life-sustaining treatment: A moral algorithm. *JAMA.* 2000;283(8):1065–1067.

33. Kagawa-Singer M, Blackhall L. Negotiating cross-cultural issues at the end of life: "You got to go where he lives." *JAMA.* 2001;286(23):2993–3001.

34. Koenig B, Gates-Williams J. Understanding cultural differences in caring for dying patients. *Western Med J.* 1995;163:244–249.

Part 3
Psychological and Spiritual Needs

8
Redefining Hope for the Terminally Ill
Debra Parker Oliver

> Those who have the strength and love to sit with a dying patient in the silence that goes beyond words will know that this moment is neither frightening nor painful, but a peaceful cessation of the functioning of the body. Watching a peaceful death of a human being reminds us of a falling star: one of the million lights in a vast sky that flares up for a brief moment only to disappear into the endless night forever. To be a therapist to a dying patient makes us aware of the uniqueness of each individual in this vast sea of humanity.
>
> —Elisabeth Kübler-Ross, "Therapy with the Terminally Ill"[1]

Although Kübler-Ross recognized the peace that comes to the dying and the rewards experienced by those working with them, society still struggles to understand how anything positive can be experienced once death is imminent. American culture does not believe hope is possible for those who know they are dying. Family members and significant others worry that the dying will give up all hope if they know they are on the verge of death. Professionals understand the importance of hope, but do not always understand how to help the dying find it in the light of impending death. In this essay I will identify the opportunities that exist for the redefining of hope for the terminally ill. This essay recognizes that hope is entrenched in meaning, and meaning is socially constructed, so there is an opportunity for caregivers to assist the dying in finding peace and experiencing the brightness that radiates before a star falls.

Every day in every community, people die. Death is the natural end of life; it happens to every person and is unavoidable, yet it remains a taboo subject. Americans, in particular, hesitate to acknowledge aging and are certainly reluctant about consciously facing this inevitable outcome. They do not face it well. Medical institutions, the places in which most people do their dying, often fail in managing the dying experience. Worse, with regard to end-of-life issues, medical practices are in conflict with societal desires and values. The hospice movement, an alternative to traditional medical approaches to care for the dying, was the first effort to recognize death as natural and hope as independent from cure. Hospice redefines hope for the terminally ill.

What Is Hope?

Hope is a word used often. Yet the definition is not conclusive and rarely operationalized. As it is generally used in medicine, it refers to a desire for cure or the elimination of disease. Professionals dedicated to palliative medicine, on the other hand, realize that hope is more than cure. Charles Corr makes a distinction between *hope* and a *wish*. He notes that the former is critical to spiritual peace and coping during the dying process, and it is grounded in reality, but wishing is not.[2] Deborah Mitchell offers the definition that hope is not a belief that something will go well, but rather a belief that whatever happens will make sense, no matter how it turns out.[3]

Authors C. Fanslow-Brunjes, P. E. Schneider, and L. H. Kimmel define hope, for the dying person, as "an inner dynamic life force that helps each dying person live life until the moment of death. It can take many forms—hope for a cure, to see one more Christmas, to live through the night." Depending on the goals of the patient, these authors suggest that hope involves four stages or phases: hope for cure, for treatment, for the prolongation of life, and finally, for a peaceful death.[4] This would suggest that we must acknowledge its dynamic and ever-changing focus for each individual. Thus, hope can be changed, re-aligned, refocused, and redefined.

Hope is defined here as a positive expectation for mean-ing attached to life events. This definition acknowledges a positive ideology, nullifying the idea of "false hope." Wheth-er what is hoped for can actually be achieved is irrelevant. Hope lies in meaning that is attached to life, not in events themselves. This recognizes that individuals can shape their hopes by finding new meanings for living. It allows a form of control over events in life that feel uncontrollable and gives purpose, allowing individuals to be active par-ticipants in the social world rather than passive recipients of life events, vulnerable to others' definitions and meanings. Thus, as long as there is meaning, there is hope. The key to hope lies in meaning, not in life events. The process of dy-ing is an opportunity to discover new meanings, not a dark death sentence, void of meaning and value.

Death in America is seen as unnatural, and it is often viewed as the enemy of medicine. America is a "death-denying" culture.[5] In 1963, Herman Feifel reported that "death is a taboo subject in the United States, surrounded by disapproval and shame. . . . [I]llness and death are considered not just bad fortune but imply overtones of personal failure and loss of status and identity."[6] The goal has been to fight death at all costs. As a result, the lines between life and death have become blurred. Ethical and legal dilemmas have pushed Americans to rethink the goals of medicine. Longer life spans and the war against disease and death have led us to reframe living, to real-ize that life at all costs may not be life worth living at all. Hope must be found elsewhere, in quality of living rather than in living longer.

The Innovation of Hospice

Until recently, the place within medicine that embraced death and focused on helping those in need near the end of life was hospice. In the United Kingdom, hospice is an actual place, a residence where the dying reside. When hospice came to the United States, it was taken as a concept and philosophy rather than a place. In this country, most hospice care occurs in the home of an individual. This home may be a personal residence or an institution, such as a nursing home. While a few hospice houses have been built in the United States, the majority of care remains in individual homes. Hospice in the United States is a philosophy of care and is delivered by a group of interdisciplinary professionals and volunteers. It is delivered wherever a patient lives. The hospice philosophy is one that focuses on living until death, on comfort rather than cure.

Hospice care grew as a direct response to the impersonal nature of traditional medicine. Hospice innovators realized that no matter how great medical technology, dying and death are certainties and there is a need to assist those making the journey between life and death. Hospice practitioners devoted their careers to helping the dying. Initially, traditional medical practitioners thought the hospice innovators must be somewhat crazy, laughing at their existential focus, critical of their commitment to pain relief and symptom management. They viewed hospice as "anti-physician." Medical representatives voiced strong opposition to it during congressional hearings in the 1980s on the Medicare hospice benefit. The medical community's reaction after the passage of the legislation was to ignore hospice, hoping for legislative reversal or public apathy.[7] Despite this lack of support, the work and mission of hospice grew.

Kübler-Ross, in her book *On Death and Dying* (1969), laid the groundwork for the development of hospice care. Her work provided a psychological-stage theory of the dying experience that created an understanding of the unique needs of those going through it. Her labeling of the five stages of grief (denial, bargaining, anger, depression, acceptance) built the foundation for all future discussions on grief. She showed that we could talk to the dying and learn from them. She pointed out the therapeutic effects of talking about feelings and provided insight into how to do it.

Kübler-Ross was one of the first to identify universal concerns of the dying. She found that unfinished business and lack of hope were issues common among all those she counseled. These concerns challenged hospice to add psychosocial needs of patients to the important goals of pain and symptom management. Although unintentionally, she articulated the mission of hospice when she wrote,

> I would add that we should not "give up" on any patient, terminal or not terminal. It is the one who is beyond medical help who needs as much if not more care than the one who can look forward to another discharge. If we give up on such a patient, he may give up himself and further medical help may be forthcoming too late because he lacks the readiness and spirit to "make it once more." It is far more important to say, "to my knowledge I have done everything I can to help you. I will continue, however, to keep you as comfortable as possible." Such a patient will keep his glimpse of hope and continue to regard his physician as a friend who will stick it out to the end. He will not feel deserted or abandoned the moment the doctor regards him as beyond the possibility of a cure."

Kübler-Ross affirmed what Feifel had suggested as early as 1963: patients need to be told they are dying. Feifel identified numerous studies that showed that between 69 and 90 percent of physicians favored not telling terminal patients that they are dying. Ironically, 77 to 89 percent of patients have reported that they want to know.[9] Although there has been a shift toward more truth telling by physicians, situations of relatives being told and patients not, as well as situations of patients being left to guess the likely outcome for themselves, are reported as still common today.[10] However, medicine as a whole is beginning to become more enlightened, with training programs on the communication of bad news and a recognition of the importance of a more open awareness of impending death.[11]

A Paradigm Shift

Within the past few years, a new interest has emerged in medicine regarding care for the dying. Legal cases have gained national attention and have begged the question, what is life? Physicians, trained in and committed to sustaining life, have appeared in the news as working to assist individuals in ending it. Studies have found that Americans are not happy with how death occurs in this country, and that medical professionals are not trained in managing the care of the dying.[12] The American Medical Association initiated training programs for physicians, and palliative medicine became a hot topic for discussion. As a result, physicians began working to understand principles of comfort as well as the practice of cure. Hospice professionals began to be recognized as experienced leaders in the care of the dying and became accepted as colleagues in mainstream medicine.

This new focus on end-of-life care is opening a public discussion as well. Bill and Judith Moyers's Public Broadcasting Service series *On Our Own Terms: Moyers on Dying* not only gave people permission to talk about death, but also encouraged people to work together to find ways to help the dying.[13] The subject of death and dying is "coming out of the closet." Medicine is ready to learn, and hospice practitioners and others must start teaching. A starting point is helping people understand that one of the most important things that can be given in the face of death is hope.

Hope is a topic in ethics literature, and it is an issue shared by professionals and others interested in improving care at the end of life.[14] However, while addressing problems of hope in the light of death and the need to find ways to help patients discover it, the literature is lacking in outlining ways for professionals to work at redefinitions. Hospice professionals have been focused on this issue for years.

Hospice and the Redefinition of Hope

In the search for meaning, one can find hope. This implies that the challenge for those working with the dying is to help them discover meaning in the light of their dying. Hospice has been helping those who have been called "hopeless" since its inception. How has hospice redefined hope? What advice can be found in the practices of hospice providers? How do they instill hope?

The first step in establishing meaning and holding a positive expectation for hope involves moving the patient from a "sick role" to a "dying role." This transition is an important process in hospice care, and it occurs with the labeling of the individual as a "hospice patient" and the hospice staff's direction of what they call "the drama of dying."[15] This metaphor of a drama comes from Erving Goffman's sociological theory referred to as the dramaturgical model.[16] Goffman's idea is that social reality is constructed within society, it lies in the interaction between individuals and groups. The idea is that reality is influenced by those involved and can be shaped and reshaped as individuals interact and interpret the meanings of these interactions. The theory uses the language of the theater to describe the negotiation of meaning between all actors and the audience. In this case, it refers to the way in which hospice staff can help patients develop a new definition of their situation, a different meaning, and begin to see something that many may see as hopeless instead as an opportunity to find hope outside of cure and a longer life.

Using the theater as a metaphor, hospice achieves a role transition (from sick patient to dying patient) through the use of props, management of the setting, and the creation of a new reference group. Props might include a hospital bed brought into the home, or perhaps a bedside commode and such things as grab bars on the bathtub or special quilts donated for the bed. Management of the setting may mean turning what was once a living room into a room where the patient sleeps. The staff will try to maintain the homelike atmosphere but set things up to function and adapt to the physical-care needs of the patient. Finally, the individuals that the patient and family interact with suddenly include all the hospice staff. These professionals who understand the aspects of dying suddenly become like family as they are coming in and out of the home almost daily, teaching family how to manage the endless needs of a dying person. All of these new activities and people set up new interactions for the patient and family—referred to, using Goffman's metaphor, as a "drama." While not a real play with a script, it becomes a dramatic adventure where interactions and day-to-day life take on a theaterlike quality. New language and meanings are negotiated, and a new reality is developed.

This does not infer that hope can be redefined only for those labeled "hospice patient." However, acceptance of the identity brings new expectations and creates a reference group to assist in the reformulation of meanings. Hospice surrounds the patient with people who acknowledge and value the new identity, often protecting the dying person from those who see the situation as meaningless and hopeless. Hospice plays an important role by creating opportunities for the family to participate in the drama, thus giving them new hope as well. The challenge for other palliative-care practitioners is to create a similar role and to provide a reference group to support the drama and its resulting meanings.

The redefinition of hope begins with those surrounding the patient: it is important not only for the patient, but for the health-care providers and family as well. One of the successes of hospice is that, from the moment of the patient's entrance, dying stands in direct contrast to previous experiences, and thus new meanings and expectations are instantly established. While sympathetic to the needs of the patients, hospices do not present this situation as sad, but rather as an opportunity, one with promise. Old meanings attached to images of technologies, physician office visits, and curative attempts to restore health are replaced with images of comfort, family, choices, and decision making. This honest, open discussion is most often met with relief by patients and families as they realize they no longer must participate in a drama where the patients are not fulfilling their role, they are not "getting well."

It is important that caregivers recognize that, as the focus of hope shifts, wishes for cure need not be eliminated. Wishing and praying for a miracle cure need not be lost when hope is directed toward comfort and dying well. Miracles happen, and there is nothing wrong with wishing and praying for them. However, people must be helped to move on with their lives with new meanings that are not dependent on miracle cures.

Finding Opportunities for New Hope, Meaning, and Purpose

An initial assessment of a dying person's fears provides an opportunity to discover hope. The two ideas, hope and fear, are interconnected.[17] Identification of fears for the dying person and a discussion of them allow an opportunity to assure the patient that his or her fears can be handled and managed in such a way that the dying person has nothing to fear. For example, if a person is fearful of pain, hope will involve the successful management of pain. This can be reinforced with promises by the physician (and nurses) to address pain issues, provide education on the management of care and medication, and to control pain. Likewise, if a patient is fearful of approaching dependency, finding ways to maintain independence and control can instill hope and help overcome this concern. Meaning is found as fears are eased through planning and education by the caregiving team.

Physicians can provide another opportunity for hope. Deborah Mitchell suggests that they make three promises to dying patients and families. First is the promise that patients do not have to die alone. In tamping down the fear of abandonment, this assurance gives those around the patient meaning for their participation in the drama and gives the patient meaning in continuing social relationships. The second promise physicians can give is that no extraordinary means will be used to prolong life. This acknowledges the importance of human interactions and touch in place of machines and life-saving technology. Meaning shifts from one based on quantity to one based on quality. Finally, Mitchell suggests physicians can promise patients that they will be remembered. This provides meaning for the life they have lived and allows them to continue to have purpose by shaping those memories in the time that still lies ahead.[18] Believing that one's sense of self is not gone, but is still under construction, allows patients a chance to reflect on who they are and how they will be remembered. The creation of a legacy provides important meaning during the dying process. These three promises begin the process of helping dying people find new meaning. Although any member of the caregiving team can make these promises, the gift of them from a physician carries additional credibility, legitimation, and validation.

Assistance with an inventory of key relationships provides yet another opportunity to establish new meaning and purpose. Understanding and evaluating them can lead patients to new goals and hopes. This sets an agenda for the possible repair of broken or damaged relationships, as well as control and management of them during the dying process, and it formulates an inventory of unfinished business to complete before death. Ira Byock notes that there are five things that need to be said to repair fractured relationships: "Forgive me," "I forgive you," "Thank you," "I love you," and "Good-bye."[19] Exploring opportunities to rebuild or enhance relationships gives life essential meaning, no matter its length. Hope is connected to the interaction between individuals, rather than to future events. Hope becomes tied to today, not tomorrow.

Assessment of an individual's spiritual perceptions gives hospice staff yet another opportunity for a discussion of hope. Many spiritual belief systems hold hope of happiness and peace for the patient and family. A promise of life after death is an important one. Even without a history of alignment with a specific religious dogma, doctrine, or creed, a dying person will usually enter a spiritual journey in a quest for meaning during this unique phase of life. Spiritual issues have been found to be the most common topic of discussion among hospice patients.[20] Spirituality offers the hope for living on in the world through established legacies, memories, traditions, and rituals. These discussions, in fact, tie the living to the dying, and the dying to those who have died before them. A search for peace and understanding through spirituality offers important opportunities for hope.

Often, the quest for hope is easily fulfilled simply by asking a dying person what they want most at this time and creatively helping them find ways to achieve it. While travel may be out of the question, other strategies can bring the destination to the dying person. Perhaps the book they always thought they would write is no longer possible, but the making of a video or audio tape to record their thoughts, experiences, and knowledge might serve as a substitute. Helping patients and families work toward the recognition and achievement of goals builds hope and creates a way to live until they die. And beyond that, the completion of these goals may leave an important gift of hope behind for loved ones as they search for meaning following the death of their family member.

An important task for those who work with the dying is to understand the emotional needs of the dying person in order to know what gives meaning to that individual. Once we understand the source of meaning for an individual, we have found the key to helping the person find hope as he or she turns from cure to comfort. Asking the patient to talk about what has given meaning in the past can help him or her verbalize feelings that lead to meanings in the present situation. Using past goals, achievements, or even frustrations to find new opportunities is yet another strategy to reframe meaning and hope.

Table 8.1 identifies possible intervention strategies that may be explored by caregivers as they seek to help dying patients. It suggests ways to assess a dying person's system of meaning and to explore opportunities to assist him or her in redefining hope from the past experience of treatment toward cure to the current reality of impending death. These assessment factors and intervention strategies are outlined in an effort to assist those working with the terminally ill in helping them find new meanings and develop new coping skills.

Table 8.1. Summary of Intervention Strategies for Assisting the Dying to Redefine Hope

1. Surround dying patients with caregivers who can find opportunity and meaning in this process.

2. Address the fears of dying patients by encouraging specific activities as part of care plans designed to manage fears, educating them regarding these plans, and expressing a commitment to fear management.

3. Work with the physician to promise dying patients that they do not need to die alone, that living will not be artificially prolonged, yet they will be kept comfortable, and that they will be remembered.

4. Work with patients on mending damaged relationships, saying good-bye, forgiving, and expressing their feelings.

5. Utilize spiritual resources to facilitate the development of meaning and the creation or implementation of important rituals and traditions.

6. Work with dying patients to achieve their goals: ask them what they most want, and work creatively toward helping them get it.

7. Utilize past experiences and systems of meaning to understand values and reinforce coping skills for patients.

Conclusion

In concluding, hope—for the living or for the dying—is an experience tied to meaning. Individuals interact with one another to construct meaning. This interaction provides an important opportunity to work with the dying and to help them discover hope once cure for their disease is not feasible. We can assist patients by understanding and addressing fears about their death, working with physicians to establish new promises, surrounding the dying with hopeful support, helping them take an inventory of relationships, tapping into their spirituality, and allowing them a safe environment to establish their own goals and meanings. We would do well to remember the words of Victor Richards, who pointed out that "the quantity and quality of care that a dying patient receives are powerful adjuvants to the growth of hope, of openness to whatever future may be his."[21]

Notes

1. Kübler-Ross, E. Therapy with the terminally ill. In: Shneidman ES, ed. *Death: Current Perspectives.* Palo Alto, CA: Mayfield Publishing; 1980.

2. Corr C. A task-based approach to coping with dying. *Omega: J Death and Dying.* 1991;24(2):81–94.

3. Mitchell DR. The "good" death: Three promises to make at the bedside. *Geriatrics.* 1997;52(8):91–92.

4. Fanslow-Brunjes C, Schneider PE, Kimmel LH. Hope: Offering comfort and support for dying patients. *Nursing.* 1997;27(3):54–57.

5. Aries P. *Western Attitudes toward Death: From the Middle Ages to the Present.* Baltimore: John Hopkins University Press; 1974; Kübler-Ross E. *On Death and Dying.* New York. Macmillan; 1969.

6. Feifel H. Death. In: Farberow N, ed. *Taboo Topics.* New York: Atherton Press; 1963.

7. Thalhuber, WH. Overcoming physician barriers to hospice care. *Minnesota Med.* 1995;78(2):18–22.

114   Care of the Dying Patient

8. Kübler-Ross E. *On Death and Dying*. New York. Macmillan; 1969.

9. Feifel H. Death. In: Farberow N, ed. *Taboo Topics*. New York: Atherton Press; 1963.

10. Thalhuber, WH. Overcoming physician barriers to hospice care. *Minnesota Med*. 1995;78(2):18–22.

11. Seale C. *Constructing Death: The Sociology of Death and Bereavement*. Cambridge: Cambridge University Press; 1998.

12. The SUPPORT Principal Investigators. A controlled trial to improve care for seriously ill hospitalized patients: The Study to Understand Prognosis and Preferences for Outcomes and Risks of Treatments (SUPPORT). *JAMA*. 1995:274(20):1591–1598.

13. Moyers B, Moyers J. *On Our Own Terms: Moyers on Dying*. Produced by Public Affairs Television, Inc.; presented by the Public Broadcasting Service, October 2000.

14. Christopher M. My mother's gift: The link between honesty and hope. *Bioethics Forum*. 1999:15(1):5–13.

15. Parker-Oliver D. The social construction of a dying role: The hospice drama. *Omega: J Death and Dying*. 2000;40(4):19–38.

16. Goffman E. *The Presentation of Self in Everyday Life*. Woodstock, NY: Overlook Press; 1959, 1973.

17. Latansi-Licht M. *The Hospice Choice in Pursuit of a Peaceful Death*. New York: Fireside Books; 1997.

18. Mitchell DR. The "good" death: Three promises to make at the bedside. *Geriatrics*. 1997;52(8):91–92.

19. Byock I. Steve's story. *On Our Own Terms: Moyers on Dying Discussion Guide*. WNET New York, Educational Resources Center; 2000:8.

20. Reese DJ, Brown DR. Psychosocial and spiritual care in hospice: Differences between nursing, social work, and clergy. *Hospice J*. 1997;12(1):29–41.

21. Richards V. Death and cancer. In: Shneidman ES, ed. *Death: Current Perspectives*. Palo Alto, CA: Mayfield Publishing; 1980.

9
Spirituality and End-of-Life Care
Scott E. Shannon and Paul Tatum

Prior to the modern medical era, spiritual issues were central to care of the dying. During the fourth century AD, hospices founded by religious orders for pilgrims and travelers became centers to care for the sick. The core values of these hospices are often attributed to the Gospel of Matthew, chapter 25: "I was hungry and you gave me food, I was thirsty and you gave me drink. I was a stranger and you welcomed me . . . I was sick and you visited me. As you did it to one of the least of these my brethren, you did it to me."

With the rise of modern medicine, the focus shifted from treating symptoms to curing diseases, and secularization separated the care of spiritual issues from medical care. In reaction to the suffering of the dying that resulted from the de-emphasis on symptom care and the prolongation of life during attempts to cure disease, the modern hospice movement arose. A key aspect of early modern hospices was the spiritual care of the dying. St. Christopher's, the landmark hospice founded in South London by Dame Cicely Saunders, still emphasizes the "religious foundation" of the hospice in its Aim and Basis Statement.

The very purpose of palliative medicine is to ease suffering. Easing suffering means more than easing the physical pain of disease. Palliation of the dying person's suffering is the easing of what Saunders called "total pain"—the combination of physical, psychological, social, and spiritual pain.[1]

Thanks to the hospice movement, attending to a patient's spirituality has become increasingly recognized as a component of good, holistic end-of-life care.

Spirituality Defined

Caregivers and authors of medical literature differ on how to define spirituality. Much of the difficulty stems from trying to define it in nonreligious terms in order to be inclusive. Though spirituality and religiosity have long been viewed as distinct concepts even within religious circles, spirituality has historically been defined in religious terms that involve an immaterial component of human nature and its relationship to a deity. In efforts to be more broadly inclusive, most discussion of spirituality in the medical literature has viewed it simply as a human being's search for meaning. This definition may not be fully true to the origin of the word and its past use. It has been, however, a pragmatic definition for medicine in that it captures much of the practical essence of traditional spirituality while not excluding the nonreligious or philosophical naturalist. In their comprehensive work *Handbook of Religion and Health,* Harold Koenig, Michael McCullough, and David Larson have proposed a more nuanced definition of spirituality as distinct from religion, yet acknowledging its common relationship to religion. They define spirituality as "the personal quest for understanding answers to ultimate questions about life, about meaning, and about relationship to the sacred or transcendent which may (or may not) lead to or arise from the development of religious rituals and the formation of community."[2]

The Consensus Conference of Spiritual Care and Palliative Medicine sponsored by the Archstone Foundation recently published its report on spiritual care as a dimension of palliative care. The Consensus Conference defines spirituality as "the aspect of humanity that refers to the way individuals seek and express meaning and purpose and the way they experience their connectedness to the moment, to self, to others, to nature, and to the significant or sacred."[3]

In concert with the medical literature, this essay will use the simple definition of spirituality as "one's personal search for meaning," recognizing as suggested by Koenig, McCullough, and Larson that this often occurs within a religious context.

The Importance of Spirituality in Medical and End-of-Life Care

There is a rapidly growing body of medical literature relating to the blending of religion and/or spirituality with medicine. One clear message from this body of literature is that patients in the United States consider religion and spirituality to be important in their lives and a part of how they deal with their medical experiences. Examples can be drawn from a wide array of medical disciplines. In a 1991 study of family practice inpatients in North Carolina and Pennsylvania, 94 percent agreed that spiritual health was as important as physical health.[4] In 1997, a study of gynecological cancer patients stated that 91 percent reported that religion helped sustain their hopes, with 49 percent becoming more religious following their diagnoses.[5] In a 1999 survey of pulmonary clinic patients, 45 percent felt that their religious beliefs would influence their medical decisions when gravely ill, and of that group, nearly all felt that their physicians should ask about their beliefs.[6] In a national survey of dying veterans, their family or friends, along with physicians and supporting health-care workers, patients appeared to value spiritual concerns more highly than did physicians. The patients specifically ranked "coming to peace with God" as second only to pain control in importance at the end of life, while physicians viewed it as much less important.[7] Based on these and many other research findings, it is clear that physicians seeking to practice patient-centered care should pay attention to the spiritual component of their patients' experiences, especially in end-of-life care.

Another unmistakable message from the literature is that religion and spirituality commonly provide people with mechanisms for coping with illness. In their systematic review, Koenig, McCullough, and Larson report on at least sixty studies detailing that people use religion to cope with a variety of diseases. They state that "in certain parts of the United States, between one-third and one-half of patients report that religion is the most important strategy used to cope with the stress of medical illness and health problems."[8] One of the groups for which these religious beliefs and practices are particularly important is the elderly. It has also been noted that the amount of religious coping appears to increase as the severity of illness or distress increases. Again, these results suggest that for physicians who want to adopt a patient-centered approach to medical care, these coping mechanisms warrant attention and respectful consideration, regardless of their medical effects. As more and more studies reveal a beneficial health effect associated with religiosity and spirituality,[9] many physicians feel justified in encouraging patients' spiritual coping strategies, if care is taken not to impose or prescribe their own beliefs.[10]

Despite the overwhelmingly positive assessment of the influence of spirituality and religion on health in general, the outcome of spiritual thinking may vary among individuals, including producing negative effects for some. While many studies have shown that more frequent church attendance (even when controlled for other, confounding variables) is predictive of lower mortality, there is now also evidence that religious struggle during illness (feeling deserted by one's church or believing that God is punishing, abandoning, not loving, or powerless to help) is predictive of higher mortality.[11] For this reason, Koenig suggests the following question as part of a spiritual history: "Do your religious or spiritual beliefs provide comfort and support or do they cause stress?"[12]

For end-of-life care in particular, the belief in an afterlife may serve as a source of peace for some patients, whereas to others, the belief in a final judgment where one may face "hellfire and brimstone" can be a source of dread. Some may view death as a finality and struggle with a sense of personal meaning, while others may view death as a step in the process of rebirth or reincarnation. A review of the studies of the relationship between religious involvement and death anxiety shows that on the whole, more religiously active people have lower levels of death anxiety, but the relationship is complex and poorly understood.[13] The important issue is that each patient may react to his or her beliefs in a unique way, and the physician must address each case individually.

In clinical practice, these spiritual issues may surface in a number of different ways. Pain symptoms that do not respond to appropriate therapy may suggest a coexisting spiritual crisis. Depression symptoms suddenly occurring for the first time in a patient may be related to spiritual issues rather than an imbalance of dopamine and serotonin. Sudden refusal of medication or care may also be related to unresolved spiritual issues. An awareness of this possibility and the willingness to address such issues will prepare a physician to provide better patient care. The Consensus Conference of Spiritual Care and Palliative Medicine recommends that spiritual care be treated with the same intent and urgency as treatment of pain or other medical problems and that spirituality be considered a patient vital sign, with appropriate screening for spiritual issues.

Spiritual Assessment

In end-of-life care, where questions about ultimate meaning and individual hopes most often affect patients' approaches to their care, it is paramount that physicians develop a method of spiritual assessment. A spiritual history goes far beyond the hospital intake question about religious affiliation. It is also more than what is usually covered in psychosocial histories. The purpose of the spiritual history is to help identify how a person pursues meaning in his or her life and what underlying hopes he or she has for life. As hope for a cure is relinquished near the end of life, a patient may turn to other, equally important hopes. These might include achieving a sense of completion in relationships with family, friends, or community; achieving a sense of meaning about life in general; or "coming to peace with God," as reported in the study of dying veterans. Without some understanding of these different hopes and meaningful pursuits at the end of life, it is almost impossible to provide patient-centered care. Not having this information requires physicians to make many value assumptions about their patients' lives, which can lead to serious misunderstandings between patients and their physicians.

The spiritual assessment may be done by a nurse, social worker, chaplain, or physician. In fact, it may often be done by all members of the health-care team, and at repeated intervals. Some initial spiritual assessment should be done at the time of diagnosis of terminal illness or transition into palliative care, but it is also important to reevaluate as health status changes. The Consensus Conference recommends that all patients receive a simple spiritual screening at the point of entry into health care and follow-up assessments with any change thereafter. The conference also recommends that formal spiritual assessments after screening has identified a need should be done by a board-certified chaplain. The chaplain should respond within twenty-four hours, document the assessment, and communicate with the referring provider.

There are a number of tools available that can assist a caregiver in making a spiritual assessment.[14] The FICA history is a popular tool that takes two to five minutes to administer (see table 9.1). A nonjudgmental opening question like, do you consider yourself spiritual or religious? shows that the physician does not have an agenda. The four-question instrument CSI-MEMO is useful for exploring spiritual sources of stress and comfort (see table 9.2). Religious patients may respond to these questions with a number of issues that they might not otherwise have discussed. For patients who consider themselves neither religious nor spiritual, this gives the opportunity to then ask if there are some other aspects of life that are particularly meaningful to them or for which they entertain some future hopes. Though it may not be understood as spirituality, many people do have meaningful aspects of their lives that they hope medical care will be sensitive to.

Table 9.1. FICA, A Two-Minute Spiritual History

FAITH

What is your faith or belief?

Do you consider yourself spiritual or religious?

What things do you believe in that give meaning to your life?

IMPORTANCE or INFLUENCE

Is your faith important in your life?

How do your beliefs affect or influence your behavior or health?

COMMUNITY

Are you part of a religious or spiritual community?

How is it important?

Who do you love or who is important to you?

ADDRESS

How would you like me to address these issues in your care?

Source: From Puchalski C. A spiritual history. *Supportive Voice.* Summer 1999; 5(3): 12-13.

Table 9.2. CSI MEMO

1. Do your religious/spiritual beliefs provide Comfort, or are they a source of Stress?

2. Do you have spiritual beliefs that might Influence your medical decisions?

3. Are you a MEMber of a religious or spiritual community, and is it supportive to you?

4. Do you have any Other spiritual needs that you would like someone to address?

Source: Koenig HG. Chapter 1. *Spirituality in Patient Care.* 2nd ed. Philadelphia: Templeton Foundation Press; 2007.

In order to conduct a helpful spiritual assessment, one needs to maintain respect for a patient's beliefs. Since many answers to questions about meaning and ultimate hopes in life are related to people's religious feelings, a physician or other caregiver should be comfortable listening to such statements. This should be the case regardless of the difference between a physician's and a patient's beliefs. The process of maintaining respect for another's beliefs is facilitated by a physician's awareness of his or her own spiritual beliefs or biases. Cultivating an attitude of "spiritual humility," regardless of how "enlightened, good, right, or wrong" one believes his or her own or others' beliefs to be, also helps maintain this respect. A patient who feels safe from being judged is more likely to share his or her deepest hopes. This provides caregivers the best opportunity to tailor their care in a patient-centered manner and to avoid tensions that may result from unrealized or differing goals.

The Difficulty of Discussing Spirituality

Despite patients' desire to discuss spirituality with their physicians, many physicians feel uncomfortable discussing patients' spiritual concerns with them, and often may avoid such conversations.[15] In a study of Missouri physicians, doctors acknowledged the importance of spiritual issues, but reported that they seldom engaged patients in conversations about them.[16] Nationwide, fewer than 10 percent of physicians routinely take a spiritual history.[17]

In the Missouri study, barriers to spiritual discussions included lack of time, inadequate training for taking spiritual histories, and difficulty in identifying patients who want to discuss spiritual issues. Some physicians have cited ethical concerns about integrating spiritual discussions into practice; they fear being accused of evangelizing by discussing spiritual issues. Factors that may prevent a patient from discussing spirituality include the patient's assumption that the physician does not have time, lack of continuity or established relationship with the physician, and the patient's fear that it is improper to discuss spirituality with the physician.[18]

Despite the difficulties of having discussions about spirituality, physicians may facilitate these discussions in a number of ways. Expressing interest over time in the person's life may help develop rapport. Reinforcing the importance of spiritual coping mechanisms shows that it is safe to discuss these issues with the physician. Also, a home visit or hospital bedside visit may be a particularly meaningful time to discuss spiritual themes.[19] Approaching these conversations in a sensitive manner, as one would any other personal issue in the medical interview, should alleviate most of the possible difficulties or pitfalls.

Intervention

Once a spiritual issue is identified, the physician may act in a number of ways. In some cases, the physician may effectively intervene simply by listening, conversing, and caring. For more formal or extended interventions, a pastoral-care referral may be important. The authors of the study that notes a higher mortality in patients undergoing religious struggle[20] speculate that physicians may have a salutary effect by referring people with such struggles to the services of chaplains. When such patients refuse a chaplain's involvement, it may be possible for physicians to contribute to their pursuit of peace of mind simply by listening to them talk about their struggles without necessarily trying to fix them.[21] Also, in the case of the imminently dying, where there may not be time for a pastoral-care consult, the physician can still play an important role merely by listening to spiritual concerns.

A physician can also enlist resources that are identified in the spiritual history. To many, a local church community is an important resource. Involving the local community in visitations and provision of communion or other rituals may be important. Care should be taken to honor the specific patient's needs. For example, in the case of a lifelong agnostic who identifies herself as a naturalist, providing a hospice room with a view to a garden may be an effective intervention.

Prayer with patients, though controversial, is an area that is clearly welcomed by some patients. In the previously cited family practice inpatient study,[22] 48 percent of patients responded that they would like their physicians to pray with them, while 28 percent found the prospect disagreeable. Because of these varying desires, even most enthusiasts for incorporating spirituality with medicine generally agree that physicians should not prescribe prayer for patients, as that may be coercive. Koenig suggests that physicians may pray with patients when the following conditions are met: a spiritual history has been taken; the patient is religious; the patient requests prayer; the physician's religious background is similar to the patient's; and the situation calls for prayer.[23] Again, this would require an individual approach that depends not only on the patient's desires, but on the physician's comfort as well. Some providers may be uncomfortable with the situation or reluctant to participate, and their position should be carefully respected.

Finally, physicians can play an important interventional role by tailoring their care to facilitate patients' being able to accomplish some of their final meaningful tasks. As stated previously, these might include achieving a sense of completion in relationships with family, friends, or community; achieving a sense of meaning about life in general; or "coming to peace with God." Ira Byock, in a paper on the nature of suffering in the context of dying well, discusses these and other potential developmental landmarks and tasks for the end of life.[24] If no such hopes have been identified because a patient is still focused on cure, a physician might also play an important role by helping a patient turn from an unrealistic hope for ultimate cure toward setting hopes on some of these potentially meaningful tasks at the end of life.

Conclusion

Spirituality and spiritual suffering are of great importance in end-of-life care. The specter of mortality almost universally causes people to raise questions and concerns about the significance and meaning of their lives. In our culture, where the reality of death has commonly been avoided, removed, or sanitized from our regular flow of life, questions about meaning and a transcendent power in the face of death are apt to come with particular force, as they may not have been deeply considered previously. Even though the physician may not be able to adequately resolve these issues, proper identification of spiritual issues, respectful listening, and appropriate referral are essential to good care at the end of life.

Notes

1. Saunders C. *The Management of Terminal Illness.* London: Arnold; 1967.

2. Koenig HG, McCullough ME, Larson DB. *Handbook of Religion and Health.* New York: Oxford University Press; 2001.

3. Puchalski C, Ferrell B, Virani R, Otis-Green S, et al. Improving the quality of spiritual care as a dimension of palliative care: The report of the consensus conference. *J Palliat Med.* 2009;12(10):885–904.

4. King DE, Bushwick B. Beliefs and attitudes of hospital inpatients about faith healing and prayer. *J Fam Practice.* 1994;39(4):349–352.

5. Roberts JA, Brown D, Elkins T, Larson DB. Factors influencing views of patients with gynecologic cancer about end-of-life decisions. *Am J Obstet Gynecol.* 1997;176(1 Pt 1):166–172.

6. Ehman JW, Ott BB, Short TH, Ciampa RC, Hansen-Flaschen J. Do patients want physicians to inquire about their spiritual or religious beliefs if they become gravely ill? *Arch Intern Med.* 1999;159(15):1803–1806.

7. Steinhauser KE, Christakis NA, Clipp EC, McNeilly M, McIntyre L, Tulsky JA. Factors considered important at the end of life by patients, family, physicians, and other care providers. *JAMA.* 2000;284(19):2476–2482.

8. Koenig HG, McCullough ME, Larson DB. *Handbook of Religion and Health.* New York: Oxford University Press; 2001.

9. Matthews DA, McCullough ME, Larson DB, Koenig HG, Swyers JP, Milano MG. Religious commitment and health status: A review of the research and implications for family medicine. *Arch Fam Med.* 1998;7(2):118–124.

10. Ellis MR, Campbell JD, Detwiler-Breidenbach A, Hubbard DK. What do family physicians think about spirituality in clinical practice? *J Fam Practice.* 2002;51(3):249–254; Koenig HG. An 83-year-old woman with chronic illness and strong religious beliefs. *JAMA.* 2002;288(4):487–493.

11. Pargament KI, Koenig HG, Tarakeshwar N, Hahn J. Religious struggle as a predictor of mortality among medically ill elderly patients: A 2-year longitudinal study. *Arch Intern Med.* 2001;161(15):1881–1885.

12. Koenig HG. *Spirituality in Patient Care.* Philadelphia: Templeton Foundation Press; 2007.

13. Koenig HG, McCullough ME, Larson DB. *Handbook of Religion and Health.* New York: Oxford University Press; 2001.

14. Koenig HG. An 83-year-old woman with chronic illness and strong religious beliefs. *JAMA.* 2002;288(4):487–493; Anandarajah G, Hight E. Spirituality and medical practice: Using the HOPE questions as a practical tool for spiritual assessment. *Am Fam Phys.* 2001;63(1):81–89.

15. Lo B, Ruston D, Kates LW, Arnold RM, Cohen CB, Faber-Langendoen K, et al. Discussing religious and spiritual issues at the end of life: A practical guide for physicians. *JAMA.* 2002;287(6):749–754.

16. Ellis MR, Vinson DC, Ewigman B. Addressing spiritual concerns of patients: Family physicians' attitudes and practices. *J Fam Practice.* 1999;48(2):105–109.

17. Chibnall JT, Brooks CA. Religion in the clinic: The role of physician beliefs. *South Med J.* 2001;94(4):374–379.

18. Ellis MR, Vinson DC, Ewigman B. Addressing spiritual concerns of patients: Family physicians' attitudes and practices. *J Fam Practice.* 1999;48(2):105–109.

19. Ellis MR, Campbell JD, Detwiler-Breidenbach A, Hubbard DK. What do family physicians think about spirituality in clinical practice? *J Fam Practice.* 2002;51(3):249–254.

20. Pargament KI, Koenig HG, Tarakeshwar N, Hahn J. Religious struggle as a predictor of mortality among medically ill elderly patients: A 2-year longitudinal study. *Arch Intern Med.* 2001;161(15):1881–1885.

21. Remen RN. *Just Listen. Kitchen Table Wisdom. Stories that Heal.* New York: Riverhead Books; 1996:143–145.

22. King DE, Bushwick B. Beliefs and attitudes of hospital inpatients about faith healing and prayer. *J Fam Practice.* 1994;39(4):349–352.

23. Koenig HG. An 83-year-old woman with chronic illness and strong religious beliefs. *JAMA.* 2002;288(4):487–493; Koenig HG. *Spirituality in Patient Care.* Philadelphia: Templeton Foundation Press; 2007.

24. Byock IR. The nature of suffering and the nature of opportunity at the end of life. *Clin Geriatr Med.* 1996;12(2):237–252.

10
The Path Ahead: Difficult Lessons for Physicians and Society
David A. Fleming

Identifying goals of treatment and expressing preferences through advance planning and documentation of it are increasingly important for patients with terminal illness, but accomplishing this is often difficult. This is particularly true for caregivers and patients of advancing age, who often resist participation in discussions about treatment options when they become ill.[1] Health-care providers also struggle with decisions in this arena. Considering limitations in treatment for patients with advanced illness can be anathema in a medical culture that strongly promotes patient autonomy and encourages intervention even when death seems imminent. Almost 60 percent of deaths in this country occur in the hospital, and of these, 74 percent occur after decisions have been made to forgo life-prolonging treatment;[2] 85 percent of all patients with cancer admitted to the ICU die there.[3] Clearly, becoming proficient at making decisions about care for dying patients is a primary area of concern for many physicians.

Deciding when and how to stop treatment is not easy because there are many unknowns. Physicians' prognoses of death are notoriously inaccurate.[4] In addition, patients are frequently ambivalent about whether they want treatment at the end of life.[5] Third, expressions of beliefs and values may not occur at a time when they can be understood by families, physicians, or others involved in patients' care, or before the ravages of illness and suffering begin to influence patients' decisions. If possible, physicians should encourage discussion with patients about end-of-life care at a time when patients are not acutely ill and when they have the time and capacity to participate effectively. The best time to do this is typically in the outpatient setting during routine follow-up rather than in the hospital during acute illness.

Caregivers are crucial to the care of patients with chronic illness and become important participants in these discussions because patients often defer to them.[6] Family members and significant others typically assume this caregiver role and represent patients to the health-care team and participate in the coordination of care. However, caregivers' awareness of treatment preferences and what is important to patients may be unclear if timely discussions have not occurred prior to the loss of decision-making capacity in patients. Caregivers who are conflicted or unsure may become frustrated and distressed when decisions must be made for their patients. Even when written or verbal healthcare directives exist, they are often difficult to interpret and may not pertain to the clinical circumstances. This frequently leads to further confusion and ambivalence for caregivers and providers who must ultimately decide for patients. Family discussions when patients have sound health and decision-making capacity encourage clarity in directives about treatment goals and the conditions of living that are acceptable or unacceptable to patients as they near death.

Physicians may have beliefs about limiting treatment that conflict with patients' and caregivers' beliefs. Physicians' beliefs cannot be avoided and should not be abandoned; however, respect for patient autonomy obligates physicians to prioritize the preferences and welfare of their patients. If doing so requires violating personal moral dictates, then alternatives must be sought to protect both physician and patient. Medical training encourages objectivism and a prudent level of detachment to encourage unbiased clinical judgment, but physicians cannot totally buffer themselves from personal feelings while in the midst of ethical dilemmas. A successful and ethically grounded physician-patient relationship is bolstered by good communication and shared decision making, which requires careful balancing of the values and beliefs of both parties.

In this chapter I will reflect on three important and broad domains of end-of-life care that may challenge the autonomy and beliefs of physicians as well as patients, and at times place them in conflict. First is a discussion on the use of health-care directives in identifying patient preferences; second, I will redefine futility as a useful concept in the modern paradigm of health care; and third, I will emphasize the importance of spirituality in the realm of health care. In each domain the subtle impact of personal belief is unavoidable and may influence the way information is conveyed to patients and how their care is delivered.

Health-Care Directives

An advance directive is a written document that tells what a person wants or does not want if he or she is unable to speak for himself or herself. The most common form of written advance directive used in health care is the living will.[7] When the advance directive identifies another person to represent the patient, the designated person becomes the durable power of attorney (DPOA) for that patient. The durability component limits the authority of the DPOA to speaking for the patient only when he or she is incapacitated—a detail that sometimes becomes blurred when the patient becomes ill but is still competent to represent himself or herself.

Advance directives are legally designed to provide "clear and convincing evidence" of a person's wishes.[8] Unfortunately, they are often difficult to apply and may contain vague language. Many physicians become frustrated by not having access to directives when needed or by patients' and families' being reluctant to discuss end-of-life issues when decisions must be made. Some have argued that the living-will concept has failed as a realistic application for health care in this country because of these concerns and others.[9] This argument tends to discount several decades of ethical concern for patient autonomy and rights of refusal, but is not without some merit when examining the data.[10]

In spite of laws, policies, and public campaigns that have encouraged written health-care directives (HCDs) over the years, only about 20 percent of adult patients actually have one.[11] This low rate of response has been attributed to many things; some people feel that they do not need an HCD, and others suspect that having one will not change the treatment they will receive.[12] As health-care choices have become more complex and medical information more difficult to interpret, few people know or can articulate what they would want in times of severe illness. Even if patients have documented their wishes, surrogates and providers often do not interpret what is frequently a long and complicated document accurately.

Physicians may resist complying with certain components of HCDs when, in their belief, life can be saved by reasonable and technically feasible intervention, such as intubation or inserting a feeding tube. Physicians often struggle with not following standard protocols of treatment, even if those protocols are contrary to patients' wishes. Fear of litigation and demands by patients' families often encourage intervention as well. Sometimes physicians are simply unaware of patient preferences: SUPPORT found that physicians knew of patients' preferences to avoid CPR less than half the time, and structured attempts to inform physicians about prognosis and patient preferences failed to modify their behavior.[13]

Resuscitation is frequently misunderstood by patients or avoided as a topic of discussion. They tend to overestimate the effectiveness of CPR and tend to want it, but for the most part they have only a vague awareness about what it will do to them or what their chances of survival after it are.[14] This may be because physicians typically do not explain it very well.[15] Preferences about CPR tend to be influenced by patients' desire for success and how their physicians convey details about the procedure and its probable outcomes. Whether they have a health-care directive or not, elderly patients tend to opt for CPR when it is presented positively by the physician, but they choose nonintervention when it is presented negatively.[16] When details of CPR and probability of survival are included in the discussion, the majority of elderly patients decide that they would not want to have it.[17] Also, patients with end-stage disease may change their minds frequently when considering quality of life and desire for resuscitation.[18]

The location and clinical relevancy of the HCD is a frequent impediment to compliance with it. A written HCD may not be readily available, or it may have been written many years earlier and at a time when the patient's values or beliefs were different. Not infrequently, the DPOA does not agree with the living will and decides contrary to its dictates. It is very difficult for family members to refrain from imposing personal values when decisions they make affect the life and welfare of a loved one. As a result, when advance planning is not done as a family and preferences are not clearly set forth, unwanted treatment and suffering frequently occur.

To avoid these conflicts, Lynn and Goldstein offer four guidelines for a reasonable strategy to improve care of patients with eventually fatal chronic illness:

- **Universality:** Enrolling in or leaving any system of care (hospital, nursing home, home care, etc.) should lead to review or documentation of advance care plans for every patient. Compliance with these plans should be a part of the quality-assurance program of all health-care institutions.

- **Continuity:** Attempts should be made to maintain the same health-care team in all clinical settings: acute, ambulatory, chronic, and home.
- **Transparency:** Documentation should be available across all settings and to all providers. The use of electronic medical records with universal provider access can facilitate this.
- **Consistency:** Emergency providers should routinely ask about advance care plans when serving patients who might reasonably be expected to have a poor prognosis or be at high risk of death.[19]

These guidelines may not be applicable across all systems, but the goal should be to provide optimum conduits for communicating patient preferences and goals of treatment within and across systems that incorporate the activities of multiple providers.

For the individual provider, it is important simply to ask the right question at the right time. Patients tend to be responsive to end-of-life questions and the advisability of completing an HCD when they have solid and trusting relationships with their physicians.[20] It is also important to encourage patients, when possible, to have discussions about values and preferences in the presence of family members, especially the designated DPOA. When all participants hear the same thing, confusion may be avoided at a later date. Revisiting the discussion from time to time will also engender clarity.

Advance directives can be a useful means of opening the door to meaningful discussions about dying. Rather than merely a prescription for action or inaction, HCDs may be the first step in encouraging useful discussions about values and what kind of life patients want to live at the end of life. In the end, it is an understanding of patients' values and beliefs that is most important in guiding decisions about withholding treatment, whether that treatment is deemed medically effective or not.

The Application of Futility

The notion of medical futility, or distinguishing between "ordinary" and "extraordinary" treatments, has been conceptually recognized for over three centuries. Medical futility is the clinical judgment that, in a patient's current clinical circumstance, it is not physiologically possible for an intervention to achieve its intended and predictable biomedical goal. But with recent decades' medical advancements, the question is no longer whether a treatment will successfully prolong life, but whether it will prolong life in a way that is acceptable. We have come to discuss this question under the heading of *futility* rather than *medical futility*. Edmund Pellegrino argues that futility is not a moral principle, but an appraisal of probable clinical effectiveness, patient benefit, and patient burden in the determination of what, if any, treatments should be used.[21]

Futility as an argument for limiting treatment is a relatively new concept for modern medicine. It was unrecognized in medical literature until 1987. Prior to the 1980s, the ability to sustain life in the face of serious illness was much more limited. Subsequently, rapidly advancing developments in medical technology and the sophistication of intensive-care units have provided the capability of keeping patients alive almost indefinitely. In the wake of the technology movement, patients and physicians began voicing concern that many patients were being kept alive well beyond the end of an expectation for a reasonably good quality of life. Out of the bioethics movement of the 1970s and 1980s, a demand for greater patient autonomy in health care represented a desire to protect and empower patients to refuse unwanted treatment, especially when it was felt to be futile.[22] This is a more expansive definition of futility that extends beyond considerations of medically effective or ineffective treatment.

With time, however, the ability to identify medical futility has blurred. In 1995, 134 articles were published in the medical literature dealing with futility, but by 1999, this number had dwindled to only 31. Many have argued that the concept of futility is indefinable and no longer pertains in modern health care. This argument is difficult to refute because there is no agreement in the medical community as to the underlying principles that determine futility. In a more practical sense, it is difficult to claim futility when medical science has the ability to effectively replace multiple organ systems that have failed.

Another difficulty with futility is that there are conflicting opinions about suffering and the value of life. Personal value judgments are unavoidable, including those made by physicians, and may influence decisions in a direction not necessarily consistent with patients' stated preferences, even if HCDs or valid surrogates are available. The difficulty lies in rating the importance of values in the futility calculus.

Pellegrino offers a morally appropriate use of the concept of futility in the clinical setting which can be useful in ethical considerations of withholding or withdrawing treatment. The Pellegrino model is a prudent guide incorporating both subjective and objective criteria that can be used in the joint determination of futility by physicians and patients or their surrogates. Unlike medical futility alone, Pellegrino's futility calculus is a proportionality equation that strikes a balance between three criteria: *effectiveness*, *benefit*, and *burden*.[23]

Clinical effectiveness is an objective determination made by the physician and is evidence based. Pellegrino's *effectiveness* takes into consideration prognosis and the probability of attaining an intended, measurable clinical outcome that will make a difference in morbidity, mortality, or functionality.

Benefit refers to what the patient perceives as valuable and is directly related to his or her personal treatment goals. It centers on the patient's assessment of "good," which is to say those goals and values that relate to whether further treatment is worthwhile or not. The patient's surrogate, in order to be valid as a surrogate, should also represent these values and goals of treatment when the patient can no longer do so. In most circumstances, the emotionality of the moment makes it very difficult for surrogates, typically family members, to remain objective and selectively represent the patient, especially when they do not agree with the patient's expressed wishes. Personal opinions and beliefs not infrequently come into conflict.

Burden is also a subjective assessment made by the patient and may refer to physical, emotional, fiscal, or social costs imposed by treatment. Burden and benefit are not readily quantifiable because of the subjective as well as objective nature of the determination and the outcomes that may or may not be acceptable to the patient. Though the physician may help to inform benefit and burden with objective facts and prognoses, it is the patient, or the surrogate, who makes the final assessment. The ultimate algorithm takes into account the proportional relationship of these variables.

Futility is therefore not a singular mathematical calculation of facts or an assessment of technological effectiveness, but a longitudinal, patient-centric, and fluid analysis of proportional benefit when treatment is questionable. The patient-centered futility model offers a means of viewing medical intervention proportionately to the needs and desires of the patient, but this algorithm should be used cautiously. Applied too rigorously, a futility determination may ignore the obligation to help the patient live the last days of his or her life as serenely and in as dignified a manner as possible.[24] The fulfillment for the patient and family of sharing one last family gathering may be well worth the discomfort of one more day on the ventilator.

Families may also demand that "everything be done" even when the treatment demanded is no longer rational. Ethically, such demands cannot be supported because they would force physicians to practice irrational medicine. Respect for patient autonomy dictates that the patient has the right to request and refuse treatment, but the right to choose is not an absolute right to demand treatment that is ineffective or morally reprehensible to the physician and the health-care team. Patient autonomy cannot override conscious moral objections or professional responsibilities to practice evidence-based medicine and uphold standards of care. In Pellegrino's words, "Beneficence and autonomy must be mutually re-enforcing if the patient's good is to be served, if the physician's ability to serve that good is not to be compromised, and if the physician's moral claim to autonomy and the integrity of the whole enterprise of medical ethics are to be respected."[25]

Patients are not ethically justified in expecting physicians to provide treatments proven to be medically ineffective or to do things that they believe are morally reprehensible. Health-care providers as persons are also entitled to respect. The nature of the provider-patient relationship, which is the moral grounding of medicine, requires that neither physician nor patient be ethically empowered to impose his or her will on the other. Ultimately, a parting of ways may be necessary if a conflict is irreconcilable. When professional and moral commitments become incompatible, a respectful separation accomplished by safely transferring care of the patient to another provider or health-care facility may be necessary.[26]

Spirituality in End-of-Life Care

Increasingly important to patients is the spiritual dimension of healing, which patients are often drawn to near the end of life.[27] Most patients welcome an opportunity to discuss faith and religious belief with their physicians.[28]

However, there continues to be disagreement as to the extent to which physicians should engage in discussions about these topics at the bedside. Many physicians are uncomfortable doing this, and some clerics feel that these issues should be left to the experts.[29]

Physicians may be uncomfortable dealing with spiritual issues for several reasons. Medical training encourages professional detachment for the sake of objectivity. As a result, physicians tend to suppress personal feelings and beliefs in the interest of unencumbered clarity in clinical judgment. Respect for patient autonomy also requires physicians to allow for and foster uncoerced patient choice, which might be threatened should physicians' personal feelings or beliefs become known. Personal beliefs incur personal biases, which may unfairly influence physicians' ability to think clearly and objectively when considering clinical evidence. If their carefully constructed professional facades are breached, physicians may feel uncomfortably "humanized" by being confronted with personal finitude and the realization that they too are vulnerable.

Being untrained in dealing with the spiritual realm of healing, physicians may also feel unable to meet the primary needs of patients when medical science has reached its limit. In the modern paradigm of health care, the good of patients tends to be defined in biomedical goals, and when these goals are no longer achievable, providers often feel a sense of frustration and even anger. Physicians may tend to withdraw psychologically and emotionally when "nothing further can be done" for their patients.

At these times, physicians qua *human beings* must come to grips with the reality of personal limitation and the inevitability of death. The physician may ask, why me? and, what else can I do for this patient? The loneliness and desperation of losing a patient, with whom the physician has had a long relationship, can likewise cause the physician to question his or her own spirituality.[30]

Clinical studies are beginning to clarify how spirituality and religion contribute to the coping strategies of patients with severe, chronic, and terminal conditions. Chochinov, Tataryn, and Clinch discovered that a positive mind-set and a supported sense of "self" tend to have a positive impact on clinical outcomes for patients approaching the end of life.[31] Now there is indication that spirituality may promote longevity, protect against cardiovascular disease, and improve recovery from acute illness.

There is little doubt that spirituality is important to patients. Many studies have shown that strong faith has a positive impact on health and well-being[32] and that people who attend church regularly tend to live longer, be less depressed, and lead healthier lifestyles.[33] An extensive review of the literature by Post, Puchalski, and Larson indicates that patient expressions of spirituality and religious belief are important to health outcomes and that recognition of these expressions by physicians, with appropriate response, is also important.[34] In a recent study, geriatric patients who reported greater spirituality, but not necessarily greater religiosity, were more likely to appraise their health status as good.[35]

Among physicians, attitudes about incorporating spirituality into the more secular art of medicine and healing are mixed, and the debate is whether physicians should ever discuss spirituality or pray with their patients.[36] A recent study revealed religious belief to be more prevalent among the general population than among physicians.[37] Those physicians who do report regularly addressing spiritual issues with patients say they do so because of the importance of spirituality in their own lives and because of the evidence supporting the connection between spirituality and health.[38] Others argue that "separation of church and medicine" should be maintained because of the broad pluralism of secular beliefs, values, and religions that exists in society and the danger of misunderstandings and offensiveness should physicians attempt to become spiritually involved with patients of different belief systems.[39]

There is no easy answer to this question. As always, when the clinical path is not clear, health-care providers must rely on their own considered judgment in finding a prudent course of action. Spiritual belief and need have always been at the bedside. Team members' being prepared and able to meet these needs, either directly and personally, or through referral to others skilled in spiritual healing, is a product of the accommodations made within the healing relationship forged with the patient, grounded in trust and mutually reinforced by all participants.

Conclusion

End-of-life care is ethically challenging because of the moral diversity of individuals. In addition, physicians are now able to keep patients alive well beyond natural limitations, blurring their ability to identify when "the end of life" actually begins in the trajectory of chronic illness and creating a perhaps subtle expectation that death *can* be defeated, or at least postponed indefinitely.[40] In the midst of these gray areas, questions about limiting treatment, identifying patient preferences, and addressing the nonphysical needs of patients are but a few of the major challenges facing health care today. And because there are increasingly more people with chronic conditions, and the population is aging rapidly, physicians have more and more patients who will be facing this time of life soon.

Discussion and guidelines have been offered here to address three specific domains of end-of-life care, but there are no easy answers. As with so many questions in health care, the responses to questions in these domains will be ethically framed but different for each patient. Ultimate solutions to end-of-life dilemmas can be found only at the bedside, through relationships of mutual respect and the recognition by patients, families, and physicians that personal beliefs and values must coexist, by the nature of this relationship, and that differences and similarities must be balanced within this moral context.

I would suggest a final note of caution. Discussing personal beliefs with patients and families may inspire their confidence, but such discussions should be approached in light of the sometimes-delicate need for privacy, the clinical circumstances, and the ultimate goals of treatment. It will serve us all to remember that the personal feelings and beliefs of health-care providers deserve respect, but that patients' need to be heard must be included in the balance.

Notes

1. High D. Why are elderly people not using advance directives? *J Aging and Health*. 1993;54:457–515.

2. Block S. Psychological considerations, growth, and transcendence at the end of life: The art of the possible. *JAMA*. 2001;285:2892–2905.

3. Dowdy M, Robertson C, Bander J. A study of proactive ethics consultation for critically and terminally ill patients with extended lengths of stay. *Crit Care Med*. 1998;26:252–259.

4. Annas GJ. Informed consent, cancer and truth in prognosis. *NEJM*. 1994;330(3):223–225 [erratum appears in *NEJM*. 1994;330(9):651].

5. Chochinov H, Tataryn D, Clinch J, et al. Will to live in the terminally ill. *Lancet*. 1999;354:816–819.

6. Fleming D. The burden of caregiving at the end of life. *Missouri Med*. 2003;100(1):82–86.

7. Emanuel E, Emanuel L. Living wills: Past, present, and future. *J Clin Ethics*. 1990;1:9–19.

8. *Cruzan v. Director, Missouri Dept of Health*, 110 S. Ct. 284 (1990).

9. Fagerlin A, Schneider C. Enough: The failure of the living will. *Hastings Center Report*. 2004;34(2):30–41.

10. Fleming D. A global perspective on healthcare decisions at the end of life. *Reg Affairs Focus*. 2001;(October):14–18.

11. Emanuel L. Advance directives for medical care: Reply. *NEJM*. 1991;325:1256; High D. Why are elderly people not using advance directives? *J Aging and Health*. 1993;54:457–515.

12. Dowdy M, Robertson C, Bander J. A study of proactive ethics consultation for critically and terminally ill patients with extended lengths of stay. *Crit Care Med*. 1998;26:252–259.

13. The SUPPORT Principal Investigators. A controlled trial to improve care for seriously ill hospitalized patients: The Study to Understand Prognosis and Preferences for Outcomes and Risks of Treatments (SUPPORT). *JAMA*. 1995;274(20):1591–1598.

14. Coppola M, Danks J, Ditto P, et al. Perceived benefits and burdens of life-sustaining treatments: Differences among elderly adults, physicians, and young adults. *J Ethics Law and Aging*. 1998;4(1):3–13.

15. Fagerlin A, Schneider C. Enough: The failure of the living will. *Hastings Center Report*. 2004;34(2):30–41.

16. McNeil B, Pauker S, Sax H, et al. On the elicitation of preferences for alternative therapies. *NEJM*. 1982;306:1259–1262; High D. Why are elderly people not using advance directives? *J Aging and Health*. 1993;54:457–515.

17. Walker R, Schanwetter R, Kramer D, Robinson B, et al. Living wills and resuscitation preferences in an elderly population. *Arch Intern Med*. 1995;155:171–175; Murphy D, Mulcahy R, et al. The influence of the probability of survival on patients' preferences regarding cardiopulmonary resuscitation. *NEJM*. 1994;330(8):545–549.

18. Chochinov H, Tataryn D, Clinch J, et al. Will to live in the terminally ill. *Lancet*. 1999;354:816–819.

19. Lynn J, Goldstein N. Advance care planning for fatal chronic illness: Avoiding commonplace errors and unwarranted suffering. *Ann Intern Med*. 2003;138:812–818.

20. Chaitin E, Stiller R, Jacobs S, et al. Physician-patient relationship in the intensive care unit: Erosion of the sacred trust? *Crit Care Med*. 2003;31(5 Suppl):S367-S372.

21. Pellegrino E. Decisions at the end of life: The use and abuse of the concept of futility. http://www.uffl.org/vol10/pellegrino10.pdf.

22. Jonsen A. *The Birth of Bioethics*. New York: Oxford University Press; 1998.

23. Pellegrino E. Decisions at the end of life: The use and abuse of the concept of futility. http://www.uffl.org/vol10/pellegrino10. pdf; Pellegrino E. Decisions to withdraw life-sustaining treatment: A moral algorithm. *JAMA*. 2000;283(8):1065–1067.

24. Pellegrino E. Decisions at the end of life: The use and abuse of the concept of futility. http://www.uffl.org/vol10/pellegrino10.pdf.

25. Pellegrino E. Patient and physician autonomy: Conflicting rights and obligations in the physician-patient relationship. *J Cont Health Law and Policy*. 1994;10:47–68.

26. Pellegrino E. Decisions at the end of life: The use and abuse of the concept of futility. http://www.uffl.org/vol10/pellegrino10.pdf.

27. Campbell J, Fleming D. Separation anxiety between religion and medicine: Reclaiming the sacred dimension of healing. *RPP J Reports*. 2004. http://rpp-dev.missouri.edu/e-journal.

28. Ehman JW, Ott B, Short T, et al. Do patients want physicians to inquire about their spiritual or religious beliefs if they become gravely ill? *Arch Intern Med*. 1999;159:1803–1806.

29. Ellis M, Campbell J, Detwiler-Breidenbach A, Hubbard D. What do family physicians think about spirituality in clinical practice? *J Fam Practice*. 2002;51(3):249–254; Campbell, Fleming. Separation anxiety between religion and medicine. See Comments at http://rpp-dev. missouri.edu/e-journal/forum1.html.

30. Campbell J, Fleming D. Separation anxiety between religion and medicine: Reclaiming the sacred dimension of healing. *RPP J Reports*. 2004. http://rpp-dev.missouri.edu/e-journal.

31. Chochinov H, Tataryn D, Clinch J, et al. Will to live in the terminally ill. *Lancet*. 1999;354:816–819.

32. Post S, Puchalski C, Larson D. Physicians and patient spirituality: Professional boundaries, competency, and ethics. *Ann Intern Med*. 2000;132(7):578–583.

33. Kalb C. Faith and healing. *Newsweek*. November 10, 2003:44–56.

34. Post S, Puchalski C, Larson D. Physicians and patient spirituality: Professional boundaries, competency, and ethics. *Ann Intern Med*. 2000;132(7):578–583.

35. Daalman T, Perera S, Studenski S. Religion, spirituality, and health status in geriatric outpatients. *Ann Fam Med*. 2004;2(1):49–53.

36. Kalb C. Faith and healing. *Newsweek*. November 10, 2003:44–56.

37. Sulmasy D. *The Healer's Calling: Spirituality for Physicians and Other Health Care Professionals*. New York: Paulist Press; 1997.

38. Ellis M, Campbell J, Detwiler-Breidenbach A, Hubbard D. What do family physicians think about spirituality in clinical practice? *J Fam Practice*. 2002;51(3):249–254.

39. Scheurich N. Reconsidering spirituality and medicine. *Academic Med*. 2003;78(4):356–360.

40. High D. Why are elderly people not using advance directives? *J Aging and Health*. 1993;54:457–515.

Notes on the Contributors

Clay M. Anderson, MD, FACP, is Associate Professor of Clinical Medicine in the Department of Internal Medicine, University of Missouri School of Medicine, and is Director of the Missouri Palliative Care Program. He also has faculty appointments in the University of Missouri Center for Health Ethics as a clinical ethicist and in the Sinclair School of Nursing as a teacher and research collaborator and is a part-time Senior Medical Director for Hospice Compassus, Inc.–Columbia Office. He is board certified in palliative care, medical oncology, and internal medicine, and leads his team in caring for people and families living with life-limiting illnesses of many kinds. He teaches and generates original work for the University of Missouri School of Medicine, University of Missouri Health Care, and beyond in the areas of end-of-life care, hospice and palliative care, pain management, palliative/supportive oncology, patient physician communication, narrative medicine, and spirituality and health care. His education includes an undergraduate degree from the University of Missouri, an MD degree from Stanford University, and postgraduate training from the University of Colorado in Denver and the University of Texas–M. D. Anderson Cancer Center in Houston. He has been on the faculty in the School of Medicine since 1997. He lives in Columbia with his wife, Michelle, and their three children and enjoys reading, fly fishing, duck hunting, camping, hiking, cooking, wine tasting, and playing games with his family. He is active in his church home in Columbia, Calvary Episcopal Church.

David A. Fleming, MD, MA, is Professor and Chairman of the Department of Internal Medicine and Director of the University of Missouri Center for Health Ethics at the University of Missouri School of Medicine. He served as a U.S. Department of Health and Human Services primary care research fellow at the Center for Clinical Bioethics at Georgetown University from 1999 to 2001. His academic career is balanced by having practiced internal medicine and geriatrics for nearly twenty years in a small rural community. Dr. Fleming's primary areas of research interest include health disparity, teleethics, care of vulnerable populations, end-of-life care, organizational ethics, and research ethics. He is also collaborating to coordinate a statewide ethics consortium to address the ethical issues of pandemic response.

John C. Hagan III, MD, is a Fellow of the American College of Surgeons. He is Editor of *Missouri Medicine* medical journal and is a two-time winner of the Ranly Award for best state medical writing. He is a graduate of the University of Missouri and Loyola Stritch Medical School, and did his residency at Emory University in Atlanta. He has published over 120 articles in peer-reviewed journals, served as president of his state specialty association, and is the 2010 President of the Metropolitan Medical Society of Greater Kansas City.

David R. Mehr, MD, MS, is Professor and Director of Research in the Department of Family and Community Medicine and Director of the Fellowship in Geriatric Medicine at the University of Missouri School of Medicine. He graduated from the University of California at Santa Cruz, received his MD degree from the University of California at San Francisco, and earned an MS degree from the University of Michigan (completed during a fellowship in geriatric medicine). He is board certified in Family Medicine and Geriatric Medicine. He was a visiting scholar for a year at the VU University Medical Center in Amsterdam. Dr. Mehr has received major federal grants from the Agency for Health Policy and Research and the National Institute on Aging as well as a Generalist Physician Faculty Scholars award from the Robert Wood Johnson Foundation. He won the Research Paper Award from the Society of Teachers of Family Medicine in 2003. He served on the Health Services Organization and Delivery study section at the National Institutes of Health, has served on several guideline panels, and is a member of the American Geriatric Society's Clinical Practice and Models of Care committee. His research interests include pneumonia outcomes, end-of-life care, and improving chronic disease care.

Debra Parker Oliver, PhD, is Associate Professor in the Department of Family and Community Medicine at the University of Missouri. She received her PhD in 2000 and her Master's Degree in Social Work in 1982 from the University of Missouri. She is former president of the Missouri End-of-Life Coalition and Missouri Hospice Organization. Prior to obtaining her PhD, she worked as an administrator in two rural hospice programs for over twenty years. She is currently researching interventions to improve hospice care, focusing on interventions with hospice informal caregivers. Dr. Parker Oliver has over sixty-five peer-reviewed publications related to hospice and palliative medicine.

Edmund D. Pellegrino, MD, MACP, is Professor Emeritus of Medicine and Medical Ethics at the Kennedy Institute of Ethics at Georgetown University Medical Center and Adjunct Professor of Medicine and Ethics at the University of Missouri's Center for Health Ethics. He has served as chairman of the President's Council on Bioethics in Washington, DC, as John Carroll Professor of Medicine and Medical Ethics, and as director of the Kennedy Institute of Ethics, the Center for the Advanced Study of Ethics at Georgetown University, and the Center for Clinical Bioethics.

Dr. Pellegrino received his BS degree from St. John's University and his MD from New York University. He served residencies in medicine at Bellevue, Goldwater Memorial, and Homer Folks Tuberculosis Hospitals, following which he was a research fellow in renal medicine and physiology at New York University. During his sixty-plus years in medicine and university administration, he has been departmental chairman, dean, vice chancellor, and president. Dr. Pellegrino is the author of over 600 published items in medical science, philosophy, and ethics and is a member of numerous editorial boards. He is the author or coauthor of twenty-three books, and the founding editor of the Journal of Medicine and Philosophy. Dr. Pellegrino is a Master of the American College of Physicians, Fellow of the American Association for the Advancement of Science, member of the Institute of Medicine of the National Academy of Sciences, and recipient of fifty-two honorary doctorates in addition to other honors and awards, including the Benjamin Rush Award from the American Medical Association, the Abraham Flexner Award of the Association of American Medical Colleges, and the Laetare Award of the University of Notre Dame. His research interests include the history and philosophy of medicine, professional ethics, and the physician-patient relationship.

Scott Shannon, MD, MSPH, earned his medical degree from Washington University, St. Louis. In 1997, he enrolled in the University of Missouri's Family Medicine Residency Program, and after graduating in 2000, he stayed at MU to complete an academic fellowship. Early in his career, Dr. Shannon developed a strong interest in spirituality and medicine. In 2005, he moved to Kenya and committed himself to improving the health of the people in western Africa. To achieve this goal, he has worked hard to develop residency training programs for doctors in the area. Because of his extensive background in health systems strengthening,

Dr. Shannon was recently chosen by IMA World Health, a nonprofit agency headquartered in Maryland, to rebuild the crumbled remains of South Sudan's health-care systems.

Paul Tatum III, MD, CMD, is Assistant Professor of Family and Community Medicine and is a member of the Palliative Care team at the University of Missouri–Columbia. He is a graduate of Southwestern University in Georgetown, TX, and received his medical training at the University of Texas Health Science Center at San Antonio. He completed his residency and geriatric fellowship at the University of Missouri. Dr. Tatum is board certified in family medicine, geriatrics, and palliative medicine. He was selected by the American Academy of Hospice and Palliative Medicine for its Leadership in Education and Academic Development program. He serves on the University Hospital Palliative Care and Ethics Committees and is Vice-Chair of the Missouri End-of-Life Coalition.

Steven Zweig, MD, MSPH, is Paul Revare Family Professor, Chair of Family and Community Medicine, and Director of the Interdisciplinary Center on Aging at the University of Missouri–Columbia. A native Missourian, Dr. Zweig is a graduate of Harvard University. He received his medical training at the University of Missouri and is board certified in family medicine, geriatrics, and palliative medicine. He also completed a Robert Wood Johnson Foundation Academic Family Practice Fellowship. His previous positions include: chair of the Governor's Advisory Council on Aging, president of the Missouri Association of Long-Term Care Physicians, chair of the Missouri End-of-Life Coalition, board member of the American Medical Directors Association Foundation, and associate editor of *Archives of Family Medicine.* He also served on the National Advisory Council for Community/State Partnerships to Improve End of Life Care (supported by the Robert Wood Johnson Foundation) and led an institutional effort to enhance training in geriatric medicine funded by the Donald W. Reynolds Foundation. Dr. Zweig has research interests in health services for older adults, advance care planning, and end-of-life care.

Index

and palliative care, 45–55;
and public's view of, 45–46;
and referral to, 1; and role
of physicians, 49; services
provided, 46–48; and
standards of practice, 51–51;
time limits for, 53; in United
Kingdom, 104

Insomnia: management of, 41
Institute of Medicine, 2;
*Approaching Death: Improving
Care at the End-of-Life*, 19
International Association for
Suicide Prevention (IASP), 91

*Journal of the American Medical
Association*, 55

Kimmel, L. H., 102
Koenig, Harold, 116, 117, 118, 124
Kubler Ross, Elizabeth, 101, 104–5

Larson, David, 116, 117, 118
"Last Acts": patient care, end of
life, 2
Living Well with Fatal Chronic
Illness Act, 64
Living wills. *See* Advance
directives
Lynn, J., 132–33

McCullough, Michael, 116, 117, 118
Medical technology: capabilities
of, 1
Medicare: and hospice coverage,
46
Mehr, David R., 68, 146–47
Middle Easterners, 88, 95
Missouri Medicine (journal), 2
Mitchell, Deborah, 102, 110
Morrison, Sean, 79
Moyers, Bill and Judith, 106

National Center for Health
Statistics, 60–61
National Hospice and Palliative

Care Organization: database
of, 55; Standards of Practice
for Hospice Programs, 50–51
Nausea: as symptom, at end of
life, 10; treatment of, 33–35
Negligence: California court
case, 17. *See also* Pain: and
risks of treatment for
physicians
Nursing home: care in, 45, 46,
47, 51, 54, 59, 61, 64, 68, 73, 74,
78, 79, 104

Oliver, Debra Parker, 101, 147
On Death and Dying, 104–5
*On Our Own Terms: Moyers on
Dying*, 106
Opiates: conversion table, 13;
formulations, 13; problems
with use of, 13; side effects
of, 14, 15; use of, in pain
treatment, 12–13
Opioids: use of, 3, 4, 19, 20, 21, 26

Pain: agents for treatment of,
9, 14, 22–23; assessment
of, 11, 14–15; barriers to
control of, 9, 18; complaint
of, at end of life, 9, 10–11;
evaluation of causes, 12;
and nonpharmacological
treatment, 9; and palliative
care, 4; pathophysiology of,
10–11, 30; patients' fear of, 18;
relief of, 12, 17–18; and risks
of treatment for physicians,
17–24; and undertreatment
of, 15, 17; as universal
sensory experience, 2–3, 9
Pain Relief Promotion Act, 22
Palliative care, xi, 1, 3, 24. *See
also* Hospice: and palliative
care; Pain: and palliative care
Patients: the dying, and ethics
of pain relief, 10, 26–27; needs
and expectations of, 5, 25–26;
and suffering, 26